Editor

Peter Sýkora

SPECTRUM SLOVAKIA Series

Volume 20

Promises and perils of emerging technologies for human condition

Voices from four postcommunist Central and East European countries

PETER LANG
INTERNATIONAL ACADEMIC PUBLISHERS

VEDA

Peter Lang GmbH
International Academic Publishers Berlin 2019

Peter Lang – Berlin • Bern • Bruxelles • New York • Oxford • Warszawa • Wien

Bibliographic Information published by the Deutsche Nationalbibliothek
The Deutsche Nationalbibliothek lists this publication in the Deutsche Nationalbibliografie; detailed bibliographic data is available in the internet at http://dnb.d-nb.de.

SPECTRUM SLOVAKIA Series
Series Editor:
VEDA, Publishing House of the Slovak Academy of Sciences, Bratislava 2019,
ISBN 978-80-224-1718-1

Peter Sýkora (Editor)
Centre for Bioethics, Department of Philosophy and Applied Philosophy, Faculty of Arts, University of Sts. Cyril and Methodius, Trnava

ISSN 2195-1845
ISBN 978-3-631-77512-7
Ebook: 978-3-631-78309-2
ePub: 978-3-631-78310-8
MOBI: 978-3-631-78311-5

This publication has been peer reviewed.
www.peterlang.com
www.veda.sav.sk

This work was supported by the Slovak Research and Development Agency under the contract No. APVV-0379-12.

Contents

Foreword

Emerging technologies are defined as fast-growing radically novel technologies with an estimated prominent impact on human society in the future. The ambiguity and uncertainty of emerging technologies at the same time raise techno-optimistic expectations, as well as serious worries about possible unwanted and unpredicted negative consequences following their introduction into wider practice. And because of their radical novelty, emerging technologies also challenge various traditional philosophical and ethical concepts, established risk assessment methods, science and technology governance and policies, science to public communication and practices within and outside the medical domain. We are also witnessing growing interactions between nanotechnology, biotechnology, information and cognitive science: the so-called NBIC convergence. Emerging technologies either individually or in a converging manner promise to open new perspectives, in particular with regards to human health. At the same time, the progress in these technologies can open new horizons for interventions into human beings which go well beyond the medical domain, with the goal of enhancing human potential in lifespan, and the physical, psychological, cognitive and emotional areas.

From the beginning of the 21st century, human enhancement with the use of emerging technologies has become a fast-growing academic topic in bioethical discourse (for example, Savulescu and Bostrom 2009). However, the sphere of academic expertise is only one element in the complex system of technology assessment in modern democratic societies. The role of the public, with its understanding of science and technology, values, fears, hopes and trust in institutions, becomes a key factor which shapes how emerging technologies are accepted and how innovation affects society. Therefore, in a democratic society, public engagements, citizen consultations, public reporting and open communication are as important in the deliberation process of policy formation concerning emerging technologies, as are stakeholder consultations, academic debates, expert assessments, government and parliament.

In the post-communist Central and East European (CEE) countries, technology assessment is almost unknown. The process of policy and law formation concerning new technologies in these countries is usually the passive and mimetic transmission of international legislation (mostly EU law) without the engagement of specialist committees or professional bodies or wider public. The paradigmatic case of this mimetic character of the policy and legal transmission in CEE countries is the process of signing and ratification of the Council of Europe´s Convention on Biomedicine and Human Rights, with the additional protocol on human cloning (Millard 2010). Although at level of The EU and The Council of Europe, challenges for societies connected with emerging technologies are widely discussed, usually no corresponding debates are taking place at the national level in CEE countries.

In addition the academic discourse on various philosophical, ethical and social aspects related to emerging technologies in the CEE countries is rudimentary and mostly published in local academic journals in national languages, isolating the discourse from that which is international.

The aim of this volume is to emerge from isolation and present the view of ten authors from four CEE countries on emerging technologies and human enhancement. They analyse the topic from various perspectives: anthropological (ch. 1, 6), ethical (ch. 2, 4), philosophical (ch. 3, 5, 7), ontological (ch. 3, 6, 7), empirical (ch. 8) and legal (ch. 9). The chapters proceed from those dealing with the topic at the general level (they also may serve as a good introduction (ch. 1, 2)), through chapters dealing with particular topics on human enhancement and emerging technologies (ch. 3, 4, 5, 6), to chapters related to the debate on this topic in CEE countries (ch. 7, 8, 9).

In the opening **first chapter**, *Liminal hotspots, transhumanism and posthumanism*, Miroslav Popper places the debate on transhumanism and posthumanism within a discussion framed by the concepts of 'liminality' and 'liminal hotspots'. These originally ethnographic concepts used for transition rituals in small communities began to be understood from the beginning of the 21st century more generally in order to describe any situation in which not only persons, but whole societies appear to be in an unstable period of transformation: in a situation "betwixt and between". Popper points out the similarity between permanent liminality and transhumanism, when human is neither human nor posthuman, when existing social structures and normativity collapse to unknown posthuman ones. He warns of the danger that if in the liminal phase of transhumanism we do not reinvent new forms of order, we will then be trapped in an unstructured situation characterized by the loss of previous coordinates, without having new ones in place. Therefore he suggests "[I]n order to avoid the danger, fear and anxiety, destruction and chaos, disappointment and pain it makes more sense to actively prepare ourselves for a posthumanist liminal hotspot".

In the **second chapter,** *Prolegomena to any ethical reflection on enhancement,* Josef Kuře shows which questions we need to ask before we start to answer the seemingly very simple question: "Is human enhancement right or wrong?" Before raising the question, he first clarifies the semantics of the "human enhancement" term. Then he analyses in detail a particular case of the human enhancement project: the concept of age enhancement. And at the end, he puts several questions we have to raise before we start to think about an ethical evaluation of human enhancement, among them: Is it instrumental reason that frees us from our (natural) limitations? Is it correct that "more is better" and "unlimited is best"? Is the enhanced human a way of overcoming the human condition, a path to Übermensch (as a form of radical enhancement) or to the self (Jungian "das Selbst")? Does enhancement cause a new estrangement of the person to themselves, or does it bring them closer to themselves?

While Josef Kuře discusses human immortality within the context of age enhancement, Juraj Odorčák in the following **third chapter**, *Transhumanism and Immortality*, focuses his analysis directly on immortality as one of the transhumanist central values. After he clarifies the concept of death, he moves to an analysis of the immortality concept, and two arguments against immortality. The first argument is the finiteness argument against immortality (M. Nussbaumm, T. May). The second argument is the argument about the possible tedium of immortality (B. Williams). Odorčák argues that one form of immortality (conditional immortality) does not necessarily lead to the destruction of the meaning of life (T. May) and its values (M. Nussbaumm). The second anti-immortality argument has been developed by B. Williams. He has been inspired by the Leoš Janáček opera 'The Macropulos Case' (Věc Makropulos 1925), which was in turn inspired by the original play by Czech writer Karel Čapek, also the author of the play R.U.R. where the word "robot" was coined. Odorčak argues that William´s argument is open to criticism from a transhumanist perspective since it presupposes a prospective practical identity, but transhumanists can equally well use the retrospective practical identity concept, which does not preclude the identity of a conditional immortal person.

In the **fourth chapter,** Ivars Neiders asks himself the question: *Can we use the capabilities approach to evaluate human enhancements?* His goal is to evaluate the suggestion made by J. Roduit that the best framework for assessing the morality of human enhancement is M. Nussbaum´s Capability Approach. Neiders shows that Roduit´s proposal has serious problems, for example, the claim that the capabilities approach can be used as a guiding and restricting tool for human enhancement evaluation. According to Neiders this cannot be justified: first, because the central capabilities are not maximizable. Second, because many capabilities on Nussbaum's list are such that they cannot be affected by biomedical means. Neiders finally concludes that although the capabilities approach can provide restrictions if the distinction between capabilities and functioning is taken into consideration, it does not provide any incentive for human enhancements.

Emil Višňovský in the **fifth chapter**, *The Pragmatist philosophical view of human enhancement,* starts with the transhumanist perfectionism, as is reflected by philosophers such as D. Pearce, R. Rorty, M. A. Walker and presented by M. Sandel. Višnovský provides a historical account of pragmatist philosophical humanism which can be seen as "a precursor of or very close ally to transhumanism". Humanism was first introduced into the debate on classic pragmatism by F. C. S. Schiller as epistemic humanism. Schiller was in favour of eugenics, which he saw as the future and saviour of humanity, almost making him the forerunner of the transhumanists. He considered human nature to be a set of potentialities that could be improved. His direct inspiration came from the Italian branch of "magic pragmatism" as promoted by Giovanni Papini and Giuseppe Prezzolini in the 1920s. For pragmatist W. James, who does not believe in the perfect life, but in achieving something higher that extends beyond the person, humanism is just one part of pragmatism. Unlike James, J. Dewey rejects Schiller's conception of humanism and he sees human improvement ('growth' in his terminology) in "expansion in which nature and the science of nature are made the willing servants of human good". At the end, Višňovský explores R. Rorty´s attitude to humanisms, which for some is one of ambivalence, while for others "a deep and persistent humanism". In conclusion Višňovský points out that although pragmatism advocates 'meliorism' of human life, "it would be a great simplification to equate it with the philosophical grounding of contemporary transhumanism".

Synthetic biology is a fast-growing emerging technology, combining molecular biology, chemistry, biotechnology, information science and engineering sciences. Its aim is to design and construct biological systems not found in nature. In the **sixth chapter** *Relevance of ontological and anthropological concepts in synthetic biology*, Jana Tomašovičová focuses on the phenomenon of synthetic biology as it challenges fundamental ontological and anthropological concepts such as life and human self-understanding. She discusses the issue mostly as background to the debate about synthetic biology in the German language environment, which differs from the world-wide debate in English in paying more attention to philosophical and anthropological questions. Tomašovičova starts with the analysis of ontological status of organisms created via synthetic biology. Do we need a new ontological category for them? She agrees with the opinion (e.g. G. Gasser) that from the ontological point of view there is no difference between synthetic biology and natural organisms, and therefore a potential ontological schism is avoided. The anthropological question seems to be more complicated: If humans are capable not only of genetically altering existing organisms but also of creating completely new life forms, the question arises as to whether this will change the way they see themselves. She concludes that we cannot simply agree with the claim that new bioresearch is anthropologically irrelevant, since we cannot ignore the impact of bioscientific research on the knowledge of ourselves, which has to be reflected in philosophical anthropology.

For decades interventions into human *germline genes* were simply not an issue because no biotechnological tools were available. That has recently changed with the emerging genome editing technologies. Now it is much more realistic to imagine the alteration, or even destruction, of human nature as far as it is determined by genes. In the **seventh chapter** *Germline Genome Editing and Human Nature*, Peter Sýkora explores the argument against radical human enhancement within the Czech and Slovak intellectual context as was originally raised by Z. Sitarčikova in her book in Slovak *On human breeding: Nanotechnologies, transhumanism and human nature* published in 2012. According to her argument it is necessary to protect human nature from radical (bio)technological interventions, because humans will be deprived of the possibility to lead a good life and reach the final end of their existence (which is the understanding of God). That happens as a consequence of the destruction of human nature due to radical human enhancement. Although Sitarčikova's argument is grounded in the Catholic doctrine of natural law and final goal of human existence, Sýkora argues, in contrast to Sitarčikova, that the argument does not require the acceptance of the Catholic doctrine of natural law, or the premise of God's existence, and can be fully transformed into a secular version. Such transformation is possible insofar as we accept naturalized concepts of human nature, natural law and the natural meaning of human existence. The conclusion is that the argument that radical intervention in human germline genes may deprive humans of the meaning of life can be independent from the acceptance of God's existence or of cosmic teleological premises.

Gabriel Bianchi presents and discusses in the **eighth chapter,** *Attitudes to progressive gene therapies in Slovakia in the light of the ethical dimensions of human enhancement*, results of the empirical pilot study recently made in Slovakia with twelve focus groups about the attitudes to genetic screening, somatic gene therapy and germline gene therapy. The focus groups were composed of adults from the general population and patients who had experience of implants and other forms of progressive therapies. The results show that although both somatic and germline gene therapy were regarded with approval overall, this is at a significantly lower level than that of genetic screening. Surprisingly, the attitudes of participants who are already undergoing technological-based treatment and progressive treatment to compensate for disabilities indicate much lower support for genetic screening when compared to participants not undergoing such treatment. Further, Bianchi frames and discusses the outcomes of the pilot study according to the six ethical contexts and seven categories proposed by Allhoff et al.

In the final, **ninth chapter** *The surgeon's failure to enhance and tort liability. Polish civil law perspective*, Andrzej Girdwoyń and Joanna Różyńska identify the main challenges which the use of cognitive enhancement technologies pose for Polish civil liability. They illustrate them using the fictional case borrowed from Goold and Maslen, in which a fatigued surgeon decided not to employ modafinil (cognitive enhancement) in order to perform brain surgery on an emergency patient. The patient suffers damage as a result of the surgery and alleges that it occurred because the surgeon made a fatigue-related error. The scenario was originally analysed through the lens of a common law system: English tort law and case law. Girdwoyń and Różyńska aim to explore whether the case would be decided by a court differently if analysed from the perspective of the continental European civil law system, namely the Polish tort law. After they made a detailed legal analysis, they come to the conclusion that according to the Polish legal system, similar to a common law system, claims in negligence against medical professionals for injuries allegedly caused by a failure to use cognitive enhancers are unlikely to succeed.

I hope this volume presenting a variety of views of ten authors from four CEE countries on emerging technologies and human enhancement will contribute to a development of the discourse on technology assessment in their countries, help to make the process of national policy and law formation more active and less "mimetic", and open the national discourses to international discussion and critical analysis.

Last, but not least, the editor greatly acknowledges the financial support provided by the Slovak Research and Development Agency - Contract No. APVV-0379-12 - for the preparation of the manuscript of this volume.

Peter Sýkora, Trnava

References

Millard, F. (2010) Rights Transmission by Mimesis: The Biomedicine Convention in Central Europe. *Journal of Human Rights* 9: 427–444.

Savulescu, J. and Bostrom, N. (Eds) (2009) *Human Enhancement*. Oxford: Oxford University Press.

Chapter 1

Liminal hotspots, transhumanism, and posthumanism

Miroslav Popper

Abstract: This chapter situates the debates on transhumanism and posthumanism within a discussion framed by the concepts of 'liminality' and 'liminal hotspots', which concern the uncertain transition between known and unknown human identity and social structures. It consists of three parts. In the first part, the concepts of liminality and liminal hotspots are explained and then their potential use is considered. The second part looks at the basic ideas of transhumanism as a new philosophical and cultural movement, and the fact that humans and society are continually changing and we therefore need to constantly re-evaluate our worldviews. In the last and main part it is argued that the concepts of liminality and liminal hotspot can be a useful tool for understanding many of the fundamental issues, and for introducing ways of 'calming' the emotional response to ideas of transhumanism. Seen through the prism of liminal hotspots it becomes clear that transhumanism and posthumanism cannot be evaluated using existing standards of naturalness, ethics, and normativity, since the currently available optics may soon become outdated.

Introduction

Is our thinking about our ability to cross the boundaries of the human species based on science or science-fiction? If it is a real possibility, should we aim to prevent it by any means or prepare ourselves as best we can for the near future? What kinds of theoretical and conceptual frames are well suited to understanding and elaborating the subject of human enhancement? Transhumanist and posthumanist ideas are associated with hopes and fears for our human future and so are attracting ever greater attention. This chapter situates the debates on transhumanism and posthumanism within a discussion framed by the concepts of 'liminality' and 'liminal hotspots', which concern the uncertain transition between known and unknown human identity and social structures. It consists of three parts. In the first part, the concepts of liminality and liminal hotspots are explained and then their potential use is considered. The second part looks at the basic ideas of transhumanism as a new philosophical and cultural movement, and the fact that humans and society are continually changing and we therefore need to constantly re-evaluate our worldviews. In the last and main part it is argued that the concepts of liminality and liminal hotspot can be a useful tool for understanding many of the fundamental issues, and for introducing ways of 'calming' the emotional response to ideas of transhumanism. Seen through the prism of liminal hotspots it becomes clear that transhumanism and posthumanism cannot be evaluated using existing standards of naturalness, ethics, and normativity, since the currently available optics may soon become outdated.

1. Liminality and liminal hotspots

The concept of 'liminality' refers to the transitional stage from a known state to an unknown state, involving the removal of previous limits and the formation of new rules. It was originally used by ethnologist Arnold van Gennep in his book *The Rites of Passage* (1960/1909) to classify different kinds of rites and rituals. He noticed that in all societies people undergo a series of transitions from one stage to another (like initiation into adulthood), which are often accompanied by special ceremonies. In his attempts to generalize the ritual ceremonial patterns, he discovered a series of three interconnected states: the pre-liminal rite of separation (separation from the previous state or position), the liminal rite of transition (testing and seeking out the unknown), and the post-liminal rite of incorporation (acquiring a new status or position).

Later Victor Turner (1964) explored the liminal stage in transition rites, in which individuals find themselves 'betwixt and between' and with no status. They are caught in transition between two relatively stable states and culturally recognizable conditions. These stable states might include, Turner suggests, legal status, profession, office or vocation, position or rank, as well as the physical, mental, and emotional conditions in which individuals find themselves at that given moment. However, it is not just individuals but the whole of society that can become trapped in this ambiguous state. Turner therefore sees liminality as an 'anti-structural' condition which leads to break down, disruption, or rejection of previous social structures and presents an opportunity to create a new social order. As he puts it, 'Undoing, dissolution, decomposition are accompanied by processes of growth, transformation, and the reformulation of old elements in new patterns' (Turner, 1964, 49). Thus both individual identity and the social order are challenged and caught in a state of limbo.

Thomassen (2009) has focused attention on Turner's attempt to generalize, expand, and make use of the transitional phase of liminality, not just to describe ritual transitions in small communities but to characterize any situation that is 'betwixt and between', including those found outside anthropology. Like Turner, he sees liminality's paradox in the fact that it is at once both unstructured and highly structuring: the most basic rules of behaviour are questioned, doubted and scepticism abounds as to the existence of the world, but the problematizing, formative experiences and reformulations of being during the liminality period proper will give the individual (and his/her cohort) a new structure and set of rules that, once established, will glide back to the level of the taken-for-granted (Thomassen, 2009, 20). Unstructured liminality, then, makes it possible for new structures to be created.

Szakolczai (2009) also sees potential in the concept of liminality - conceived of as the breaking down of limits and boundaries - for exploring different kinds of events or situations, in which the old order dissolves, whilst allowing for new institutions and structures to be formed. Szakolczai takes as his analogy the initiation ceremony rituals described by van Gennep and Turner that a child undergoes when transitioning into adulthood. As he puts it, 'the child has died, but only to be re-born again as an adult' (Szakolczai, 2009, 148). Unlike Turner, however, he emphasizes that suffering may result from the breakdown of the previous stability and from potential failure in new unstable circumstances. Szakolczai considers this primarily to be because when in a liminal situation, individuals - full of uncertainty - attempt to imitate others, and at this point there is a risk that this will be abused by the unscrupulous, whom the imitators will be unable to distinguish from charismatic leaders. That is why, in some liminal situations, tyrants may come to power who are capable of turning the country into a totalitarian state over a relatively long period of time.[1]

In general, liminality can be defined as a sensitive boundary on which transformation takes place. In the human domain it means that once you cross it, you become a different person or a person with a different identity. As individuals change, so too does the structure of society. Therefore Stenner (2016) sees the liminal phase as 'a zone of becoming in the context of which normal structural rules no longer apply'. He also stresses that it is accompanied with an 'uncertainty and volatility that makes for the heightened intensity of emotionality typical in liminal conditions'. He thus proposes that, ontologically, we should think about phases of liminality 'as gaps, ruptures, and voids in structure: as marginal places and moments of movement where old structure is destroyed and new structure is created' (ibid, 47).

[1] For a more detailed analysis of the concept of liminality covering the ethnological and cultural anthropological aspects as well as sociological, social, and political ones, see Popper (2016).

The term 'liminality' implies that unstable periods 'betwixt and between' develop over time into stable states or structures. However, it may be that this transition is no longer exceptional and short term, but becoming commonplace and long term. Szakolczai (2017, 231) uses the concept of 'permanent liminality' to describe 'situations in which temporary suspension of normality becomes permanent'. In the state of permanent liminality 'temporariness' became 'steadiness'. Szakolczai (ibid) stresses that permanent liminality produces a sense of entrapment that leads to over-emotionality.

This long-term disruptive effect, accompanied by negative emotions, has been referred to as a liminal hotspot. According to Greco and Stenner (2017) the novel psychosocial concept of the liminal hotspot can be used to explore how the dynamics at play in permanent liminality mediate psychosocial and sociopsychological relations. Here they are thinking of new forms of mutual interaction between individual and society occurring in a liminal hotspot. Psychosocially, then, people have to adapt or balance their own parameters to the new structures, events, and patterns by transforming their identities, while sociopsychologically they have to work out how to cooperate and coordinate themselves in emergent, unknown dynamic situations. A liminal hotspot can therefore be defined as 'an occasion characterised by the experience of being trapped in the interstitial dimension between different form-of-process, and in the situation of ontological indeterminacy that characterises such a dimension' (Greco, Stenner, 2017, 152). If the focus is more on our emotionality, a liminal hotspot can be viewed (like liminality) as 'an occasion of sustained uncertainty, ambivalence and tension in which people feel "caught suspended" in the limbo of an in-between phase of transition' (Stenner, Greco, Motzkau, 2017, 141–142).

This chapter will demonstrate how the notions of liminality and liminal hotspots can be applied to transhumanism and posthumanism. But first a more detailed examination of the basic ideas of transhumanism is required.

2. Transhumanism and posthumanism

Although people's attempts to improve their bodily or mental states – from body decoration to natural drugs – is one of the key characteristics of our species, the scientific foundations of transhumanism can be traced back to the Age of Enlightenment. At the beginning of this age, Francis Bacon saw the potential of empirical sciences to enhance our lives. He wrote 'The task and purpose of human Power is to generate and superinduce on a given body a new nature or new natures'. Subordinate to this primary task was 'the transformation of concrete bodies from one thing into another within the bounds of the Possible' (Bacon, 2000/1620, 102).

In the humanist period Condorcet believed that one day medicine would become so powerful it could fundamentally extend the length of human life.

> Certainly, man will not become immortal, but will not the interval between the first breath that he draws and the time when in the natural course of events, without disease or accident, he expires, increase indefinitely? ... we are bound to believe that the average length of human life will forever increase... (Condorcet, 2012, 146)

In the first half of the twentieth century, ideas on human transformation became officially known as 'transhumanism' thanks to Julian Huxley, who wrote:

> The human species can, if it wishes, transcend itself – not just sporadically, an individual here in one way, an individual there in another way – but in its entirety, as humanity. We need a name for this new belief. Perhaps *transhumanism* will serve: man remaining man, but transcending himself, by realizing new possibilities of and for his human nature. 'I believe in transhumanism': once there are enough people who can truly say that, the human species will be on the threshold of a new kind of existence, as different from ours as ours is from that of Pekin man. (Huxley, 1957, 17)

In the current era, transhumanism is perhaps best defined as:

> Philosophies of life (such as extropian perspectives) that seek the continuation and acceleration of the evolution of intelligent life beyond its currently human form and human limitations by means of science and technology, guided by life-promoting principles and values. (More, 2013a, 3)

At the same time transhumanism is closely connected with the singularity, as explicitly indicated by Vinge (2013): 'Computer networks and human-computer interfaces ... could lead to the Singularity' (370). '... And while mind and self will be vastly more labile than in the past, much of what we value (knowledge, memory, thought) need never be lost' (373).

Before we can look for close parallels between liminality and liminal hotspots on the one hand and transhumanism on the other, a crucial difference has to be explained. Many key proponents of liminality (e.g. Stenner, Szakolczai) are more sympathetic to postmodernism than to modernism. Although transhumanism is a new philosophical and cultural movement that shares some common values with postmodernism, like the 'need for change, reevaluating knowledge, recognition of multiple identities, and opposition to sharp classifications of what humans and humanity ought to be' it 'seeks a transmodernity or hypermodernism rather than arguing explicitly against modernism' (More and Vita-More, 2013, 4). It stresses 'the need for inclusivity, plurality and continuous questioning of our knowledge, as we are a species and a society that is forever changing' (ibid). Many advocates of postmodernism set themselves apart from humanism, but transhumanism develops core Enlightenment ideas such as the use of scientific methods, individual rights, and the possibility and desirability of progress (More, 2013a). The idea that the internal cognitive architecture of the mind is the basis of human intelligence and rationality is very important in transhumanism. Therefore, in contrast to social constructionism, the processes of deconstructing and reconstructing reality are not centred on discovering the meanings of discourses seeking greater social justice and emancipation, but predominantly on our cognitive processes that can either be enhanced, genetically modified, or augmented using synthetic machines. The focus is on technologies that may overcome many of the current human limits.

According to More (ibid), there are two ways of viewing the philosophy of transhumanism. On the one hand 'trans-humanism', growing out of Enlightenment humanism, stresses the possibility and desirability of progress (greater cognitive capacities, more refined emotions, and an end to suffering from diseases and ageing) and that it can be accomplished by applying science and technology rather than praying for it. On the other hand 'transhuman-ism' emphasizes openness to improvement and opposition to authoritarian social control and unnecessary hierarchy. The dominant features of transhumanism can be said to be a belief in progress, both on the individual level by enhancing peoples' abilities as well as on the social level by the better organization of society as a whole. One of the crucial problems it needs to solve – how transhumanists would mediate psychosocial and sociopsychological relations – is similar to the issues addressed in the work of Greco and Stenner (2017) in exploring liminal hotspots.

In his 'Letter to Mother Nature', More (2013b) expressed the interests of several influential Extropians (people optimistically seeking to improve the human condition). Besides conveying gratitude to Mother Nature for what she has made us, his letter contained seven amendments:

> We will no longer tolerate the tyranny of aging and death ... We will expand our perceptual range through biotechnological and computational means ... We will improve on our neural organization and capacity, expanding our working memory, and enhancing our intelligence ... We will supplement the neocortex with a 'metabrain' ... We will no longer be slaves to our genes ... We will cautiously yet boldly reshape our motivational patterns and emotional responses in ways we, as individuals, deem healthy ... we will not limit our physical, intellectual, or emotional capacities by remaining purely biological organisms ... These amendments to our constitution will transition us from a human to a posthuman condition as individuals. (More, 2013b, 450)

These amendments clearly show that the basic methods of human enhancement will be nano-bio-info-cogno technology based. The last point in the transhumanist declaration (2012, 55) reads: 'We favor morphological freedom - the right to modify and enhance one's body, cognition and emotion. This freedom includes the right to use or not use techniques and technologies to extend life, preserve the self through cryonics, uploading, and other means, and to choose further modifications and enhancements'. Amendment No. 1 seems to be more important and is also highlighted by Broderick (2013, 434): 'The true goal of transhumanism is the defeat of aging and death. It is a Promethean ambition, but increasingly we see steps in that direction'.

In distilled form the seven amendments can be applied in three basic areas of human enhancement covered by the concept of *posthuman*. The term 'posthuman' refers to a 'human' in possession of at least one of the three basic capacities: healthspan, cognition, and emotion that significantly exceeds the maximum that human beings can achieve without new technological means (Bostrom, 2013). A similar definition is that by Max More who characterizes posthumans as persons of unprecedented physical, intellectual, and psychological capacity, and as self-programming, self-constituting, potentially immortal, unlimited individuals[2]. Although compared with transhumans, posthumans would be radically different forms of human beings, Bostrom (2013) uses many examples to argue that attempts at

[2] See: http://www.aleph.se/Trans/Words.

this kind of human enhancement largely grow out of traditional ethics and that societies value posthuman capacities, implicitly at least. For instance, attempts are made to improve healthspans, with medical research receiving strong support from governmental and non-governmental organizations, and people take preventive measures to stay healthy (from vitamins to airbags), attend medical facilities when they are sick, and it is usual to pay extra for risky and dangerous work. Where cognition is concerned, again society promotes both general and specific kinds of education to improve our thinking abilities and develop other specific traits and talents. People also drink tea, coffee, or energy drinks and take (natural) medicines to make them more alert especially when they have to perform intellectually. The majority of people also try (through education, training, meditation, pills) to reduce levels of aggression, sadness, hate, and fear and to make them more sensitive, emphatic, compassionate, happy, joyful, and take pleasure in becoming better beings. While none of these examples, as Bostrom (2013) acknowledges, imply an explicit desire to become posthuman, there is no firm line indicating maximum healthspan, cognition, and emotion beyond which human enhancement would not be desirable (for many people).

He also points to the paradox that many religious people who fear posthumanism believe in their own radical posthuman transformation after death and see it as desirable. The question is whether it is more meaningful to strive for this kind of transformation during our life on earth or passively wait and believe that it will be realized in heaven. Therefore Bostrom (2005) advocates rooting transhumanism in rational humanism, in which the emphasis is on empirical science and critical reason as opposed to revelation and religious authority.

One consequence of biological and cultural evolution is that continual changes in humans and society are a stable feature of human nature. Humans are not static beings living in a static environment – quite the opposite. They are capable of transforming life's conditions, of permanently trying to improve their lives by changing the outside world as well as their own capabilities, and they often find themselves in liminal situations. However, thus far the pace of change has not seriously challenged our biological constitution. In the near future, we may witness our own radical transformation to beyond our current biological limits. The aim in transhumanism is to promote human enhancement achieved through modern technologies that may substantially alter our individual biological predispositions as well as our social and ecological niche.

3. Liminal hotspots, transhumanism, and posthumanism

Searching for similarities between liminal hotspots and posthumanism might help us consider the possible future changes with greater balance and less emotion. Stenner and Moreno (2013) stress that although every actuality can be seen as liminal, some situations (like birth, death, crisis, or initiation) are more liminal than others. From this perspective, transhumanism can be seen as offering a prototype of a liminal situation, as it may radically challenge the 'old' forms of social order and identity and call for a 'new' one. During the transhumanist period we would be both human and not human, or neither human nor posthuman. Hence the focus on the concept of human nature and the critical voices accusing transhumanism of having Promethean aspirations to transform it, or the concern that 'essential' properties of our identity may be lost (see, e.g. Sandel, 2004, Schneider, 2008). This is why the very possibility of transhumans triggers affective responses and emotions linked to growing existential anxiety and new possibilities and experiences.

FM-2030 (1989) defines a transhuman as a 'transitional human'. From this, the similarity between permanent liminality and transhumanism is obvious. Framing human enhancement as a liminal situation allows us to argue that our present beliefs about people and society will soon become outdated and inappropriate and that we may be faced with the collapse of existing structures in the transformation to an unknown posthuman state. Sooner or later, as we undergo personal and social transformation, we could be in a situation requiring the renegotiation of human nature, the reformulation of rules, norms, rights and duties, and the re-establishment of social structures.

Although there are a range of ideas and clear parallels between liminality, liminal hotspots, and transhumanist ideas, the meaning of the keyword "transformation" requires clarification in order to avoid misunderstandings. For example, when Bostrom (2013) talks of the human transformation of a child into an adult during maturation, he stresses that it is accompanied by changes in cognitive and emotional capacities and involves the disruption of identity. He uses it as an analogy for the transformation of a human into a posthuman. Human maturation resembles liminality in the sense it was originally used by van Genep, who was interested in the fact that in all societies people undergo a series of transitions, such as the transition from childhood to adulthood. These are liminal situations for the participants, who move from a known to an unknown state, but from the perspective of other adults both these states are 'known'. Transformation from human to transhuman and posthuman is closer to permanent liminality in modern societies (Szakolczai, 2017, Greco, Stenner, 2017) where the rapid pace of change means existing social structures may break down before new ones are established. Therefore the future is unknown to everyone.

Germinal choice technology (GCT) is a good example of a technology whose use could lead to the emergence of a liminal hotspot. The outcomes would not only affect people today, but future generations as well. Stock (2013, 307) argues that GCT

> interventions would so change the trajectory of human life and the essence of the human condition as to render our past irrelevant to us in many ways. ... As we head down the path of biological modification, we will gradually cease to be who we have always been. If we live longer, healthier, vastly different lives, we may end up estranged from the world we now inhabit.

It is this that leads to fear, uncertainty, and insecurity. Many people have negative attitudes not just towards GCT but to many developing technologies that could alter human life. This is the biggest difference between liminality in the sense where the traditional order is suspended, which is more or less predictable, and the harder to predict liminal hotspots that would break down the current social structures and make the old order of norms redundant.

This difference in the transformation of humans and society is even more obvious when we broaden the scope to include not just human enhancement, but the enhancement of artificial intelligence as well. One view of what the dramatically changed world might look like in the near future is encompassed in the concept of the singularity. Proponents of the technological singularity suggest that rapid advances in nano-bio-info-cogno technologies will lead to radically super-intelligent entities suddenly exceeding current human intelligence, which will further boost technological progress based on a positive feedback loop. This way the singularity will carry us into the posthuman era. Vernor Vinge (2013) describes several ways in which this may happen, such as the 'awakening' of computers, the 'waking up' of large computer networks or computer-human interfaces, or through biologically improved human intelligence. Progress in technological development seems to go hand in hand with human enhancement, to some extent at least. If that were not the case, people would very soon be unable to keep apace of their own technological artefacts. Nonetheless the transformation of the current world into an unknown reality will be unprecedented. It is entirely possible that we will enter the posthumanist era unenhanced and unprepared.

Bostrom (2013) specifies three distinct theoretical entities that can be defined by the singularity: an instant of time when the speed of technological development will be very rapid, a period beyond which almost nothing will be predictable, and the creation of artificial superintelligence. Sandberg (2013) also stresses that a basic characteristic of the singularity is that it is a point in time beyond which it will be hard to predict future states; although he notes more broadly that the term also denotes steep changes in the social structure and economy caused by the use of technologies. Singularity can be viewed as the next evolutionary stage, which will shake the very pillars of our current social structures and lead to discontinuity with the past. It can be seen as one of the best possible examples of a liminal hotspot. As Vinge (2013, 366) puts it, 'This change will be a throwing-away of all the human rules, perhaps in the blink of an eye - an exponential runaway beyond any hope of control. ... It is a point where our old models must be discarded and a new reality rules ...' In this prototypical liminal hotspot situation, change will be fast and radical, the future will become almost unpredictable, and known social structures could collapse like a house of cards. Even imagining this point in time triggers rejection emotions in many people.

It seems that the singularity is not the only possibility on the horizon, although there is little doubt that technological progress is growing rapidly. At present little can be said about specific forms of posthumanism, and transhumanism is gradually emerging on the scene. The question then is not whether we will face a liminal era in connection with human enhancement, but to what degree and extent will liminality bring about discontinuity with our past and present state.

Moreover, many of the transformations in "human nature" will have an irreversible effect on our descendants, particularly in relation to reproductive cloning, foetal therapies that could alter the egg or sperm, and germline procedures, all of which are frequently rejected by experts and public alike. Stock (2013), however, argues that once these 'inheritable genetic modification' procedures become safe and reliable, regulations will determine whether attempts to clone humans or advanced germinal choice technologies enter the public domain, but not whether they occur. The same holds for any other kind of human enhancement. This argument is about the impossibility of blocking technological progress, including anti-ageing medicine, smart drugs, genetic modification, and other methods of improving healthspan, cognition, and emotions. On the other hand, many people (mainly Extropians) welcome the coming phase of the posthumanist liminal hotspot, seeing it as the fulfilment of the human dream of transcending our biological limits. Demographic trends suggest that parents in small families with one or two babies wish to raise as many successful children as they can. Therefore, as Stock believes, it is reasonable to expect that many parents would willingly make use of modern technologies to select certain aspects of their children's genetics.

Even today we are witnessing gradual changes in the value system concerning human enhancement. Miah (2008) proposes a three-value typology of human enhancement: the first type is the least problematic and is known as *engineering traits of accepted value*, which includes the fluoridization of tap water or inoculations. The second is *engineering traits of contested value* (e.g. engineering piety and patriotism). The third is extending human capacities (such as intelligence or height) and new kinds of human functions (e.g. flight, change of colour). I will now use this taxonomy as the basis for further discussing the possibilities of trans- and posthumanism.

Although the boundaries of this classification are blurred, as will be further shown, its usefulness lies in the fact it draws a line between the possibilities of (technological) progress today, in the near future, and in the distant future. As Miah (2008, 6) recognizes, 'an enhancement to height could fall within all three categories since it might 1) reduce certain risks of contracting illness 2) lead to a level of height that precludes certain life choices or conveniences, and 3) extend someone beyond the normal range of human functioning'. These boundaries could also change over time, with what was almost unimaginable in the past being viewed as common in the present. As Miah (ibid, 5) puts it 'if humans slowly developed into winged creatures, then the parameters of what is humanly possible would also shift'. It is important to stress this permanent shift in debates with opponents of transhumanism who often use as their main argument the breaking down of the boundaries of naturalness and normativity.

The same holds for the notion of liminality. What seems liminal now may be viewed as 'normal' or common in the future, as cultural evolution changes our perception of what is possible, acceptable, and traditional whilst also enriching our comprehension of nature and the world. As hormonal contraception, the cryopreservation of gametes or embryos, or in vitro fertilization gradually become standard, regular, and natural, and they will no longer be associated with liminality.

Looking at Miah's (2008) proposed typology of human enhancement through the optics of liminality, the first type – engineering traits of accepted value – is neither radical nor liminal as it reflects the gradual increase in knowledge on human health in a broad sense and technological advances to improve human life.

On the other hand the second and third types are liminal, and yet there is a great difference between them. While the second type – engineering traits of contested value – can be achieved in the medium term and many of its implications can be foreseen, the third type resembles the post-singularity era of posthumanism and its outcome is quite unpredictable.

It therefore seems reasonable to focus mainly (but not exclusively) on the second type and to try to understand how the social structures and normativity can and must change in the near future to keep pace with human enhancement. At present it seems meaningful to start solving problems associated with successive changes in longevity (like the pension system, the health and social care system, employment, leisure activities) rather than speculate about immortality and its consequences. It's worth looking at the new rules and norms associated with the enhancement of our cognitive abilities (intelligence, memory, alertness) within our biological limits (e.g. through smart drugs) rather than paying too much attention to an era in which the limits of our cognitive abilities will be extended beyond human characteristics. Somewhere here lies the blurred boundary between science and science-fiction. Science-fiction always looks ahead, offering a range of possibilities without the need to prove its visions (in comparison with science), and some of these will be fulfilled while others will never happen. At the same time, it brings us to a permanent state of liminality as it moves the boundaries every time a future state is approached. In science-fiction, reality is never sufficiently real, satisfactory, or stable; the social structures are not adequate and norms are suspended.

The liminality connected with human enhancement can be viewed from two perspectives. One deals with improving individual deficits to help people attain the highest level of human possibility. The second is about altering our current traits and skills. The first is similar to the original liminal rites of passage and is analogical to the transition from childhood to adulthood – that means that those who are 'more talented' already 'know' how the individual will be enhanced. The second is enhancing in the sense of going beyond the limits of human nature and would call for a radical change in social structures and norms. If current norms become outdated, then the existing prohibitions will also be ineffective.

If instead of lamenting over transhumanism or searching for solutions that ban all 'radical' kinds of human enhancement, we choose to prepare for the coming changes, we could lessen the risks of oncoming liminal hotspot. The sooner we start dealing with the first and second levels of human enhancement and gradually implement and test clever solutions, the better we will be able to more realistically imagine what changes level three will bring, if it ever arrives.

The demanding nature of the second type - engineering traits of contested value - can be clearly illustrated using the example of vices and virtues. Even if we knew how to strengthen virtues and eliminate vices and thought this appropriate, defining good and bad behaviour remains a problem. As MacIntyre (2007) argues virtues are dependent on a particular context and social structure and therefore cannot be judged per se. Similarly, Curry (2008) distinguishes two basic kinds of virtues: Christian (humility, meekness, quietude, asceticism, obedience) and pagan (beauty, strength, courage, magnanimity, leadership), and sees them as two sides of the same coin or two aspects of human nature. In times of peace the virtues of humility, modesty, and patience may be valued more; however, during war the virtues of power, courage, and leadership may be considered desirable character traits. If we have difficulty unequivocally distinguishing virtues from vices, or deciding whether to favour virtues of dominance over virtues of submission, then it is not clear on what basis we would engineer our children's traits, as their value may fluctuate depending on societal demands. Therefore the moral domain seems to be one of the most problematic issues of human enhancement.

Conclusion

The more prepared we are for the new reality, the shorter the period of entrapment within the liminal phase 'betwixt and between', and the less opportunity there will be for the 'tricksters' ready to occupy the empty space and entrap us in a new-age form of totalitarianism governed and controlled by new nano-bio-info-cogno technologies.

The 'unscrupulous' could misuse extreme approaches to human enhancement, be they sticking with outmoded standards or headlessly swooping into the unknown. However, this is not the only, nor the worst, possibility. In the liminal phase of transhumanism it will be up to us to reinvent new forms of order. Otherwise we will be trapped in an unstructured situation characterized by the loss of previous coordinates without having new ones in place that would better reflect the actual state of affairs. If we are not able to fulfil the task, posthumans, who may not have the interests of people at heart, will do so instead. In order to avoid the danger, fear and anxiety, destruction and chaos, disappointment and pain it makes more sense to actively prepare ourselves for a posthumanist liminal hotspot. The second option of banning potential advanced technologies because naturalness, ethics, and normativity have not kept up and crowding out research on radical human enhancement undertaken outside the public sphere seems to be much more dangerous. Regardless of which we choose, our liminal future, with all its positive and negative potentialities, is just around the corner awaiting our next steps.

Acknowledgement

This work was supported by Slovak Research and Development Agency contract No. APVV-0379-12.

Literature

Bacon, F. (2000/1620). The New Organon. In: L. Jardine and M. Silverthorne (Eds.): *Cambridge Texts in the History of Philosophy*. Cambridge: Cambridge University Press, 1–252.

Bostrom, N. (2005). A History of Transhumanist Thought. *Journal of Evolution and Technology, 14*, 1, http://jetpress.org/volume14/bostrom.html.

Bostrom, N. (2013). Why I Want to be a Posthuman When I Grow Up. In: M. More and N. Vita-More (Eds.): *Classical and Contemporary Essays on the Science, Technology, and Philosophy of the Human Future. The Transhumanist Reader*. Oxford: Wiley-Blackwell, 28–53.

Broderick, D. (2013). Trans and Post. In: M. More and N. Vita-More (Eds.): *Classical and Contemporary Essays on the Science, Technology, and Philosophy of the Human Future. The Transhumanist Reader*. Oxford: Wiley-Blackwell, 430–437.

Condorcet, N. (2012). Political Writings. In: S. Lukes and N. Urbinati (Eds.): *Cambridge Texts in the History of Political Thought*. Cambridge: Cambridge University Press, 1–205.

Curry, O. (2008). The Conflict-Resolution Theory of Virtue. In: W.S. Armstrong (Ed.): *Moral Psychology, Vol. 1: The Evolution of Morality: Adaptations and Innateness*. Cambridge: MIT Press, 251–261.

FM-2030 (originally Esfandiary) (1989). *Are You a Transhuman?* New York: Warner Books.

Greco M., Stenner P. (2017). From Paradox to Pattern Shift: Conceptualising Liminal Hotspots and Their Affective Dynamics. *Theory & Psychology, 27*, 2, 147–166.

Huxley, J. (1957). *New Bottles for New Wine*. London: Chatto & Windus.

MacIntyre, A. (2007). *After Virtue: A Study in Moral Theory.* Notre Dame: University of Notre Dame Press.

Miah, A. (2008). Engineering Greater Resilience or Radical Transhuman Enhancement? *Studies in Ethics Law and Technology,* 2, 1, Article 5. DOI: https://doi.org/10.2202/1941-6008.1023

More, M. (2013a). The Philosophy of Transhumanism. In: M. More and N. Vita-More (Eds.): *Classical and Contemporary Essays on the Science, Technology, and Philosophy of the Human Future. The Transhumanist Reader.* Oxford: Wiley-Blackwell, 3–17.

More, M. (2013b). A Letter to Mother Nature. In: M. More and N. Vita-More (Eds.): *Classical and Contemporary Essays on the Science, Technology, and Philosophy of the Human Future. The Transhumanist Reader.* Oxford: Wiley-Blackwell, 449–450.

More, M., Vita-More, N. (2013). *Classical and Contemporary Essays on the Science, Technology, and Philosophy of the Human Future. The Transhumanist Reader.* Oxford: Wiley-Blackwell, 1–2.

Popper, M. (2016). Human Enhancement and the Concept of Liminality. *Human Affairs, 26*, 128–139.

Sandberg, A. (2013). Morphological Freedom – Why We Not Just Want It, but Need It. In: M. More and N. Vita-More (Eds.): *Classical and Contemporary Essays on the Science, Technology, and Philosophy of the Human Future. The Transhumanist Reader.* Oxford: Wiley-Blackwell, 56–64.

Sandel, M. (2004). The Case Against Perfection. *The Atlantic.* Available online: http://www.theatlantic.com/magazine/archive/2004/04/the-case-against-perfection/302927/ (25. 02. 2015).

Schneider, S. (2008). Future Minds: Transhumanism, Cognitive Enhancement and the Nature of Persons. Retrieved from http://repository.upenn.edu/neuroethics_pubs/37 (17.10.2015).

Stenner P. (2016). Liminalität, Un-Wohl-Gefühle und die affektive Wende [Liminality, Un-wellbeing, and the Affective Turn]. In: E. Mixa, S. M. Pritz, M. Tumeltshammer, and M. Greco (Eds.): *Un-Wohl-Gefühle: Eine Kultureanalyse Gegenwärtiger Befindichkeiten [Un-wellbeing: A Cultural Analysis of Contemporary Feelings].* Bielefeld, Germany: Transcript-Verlag, 45–67.

Stenner, P., Greco, M., Motzkau, J. (2017). Introduction to the Special Issue on Liminal Hotspots. *Theory & Psychology, 27*, 2, 141–146.

Stenner, P., Moreno-Gabriel, E. (2013). Liminality and Affectivity: The Case of Deceased Organ Donation. *Subjectivity, 6*, 3, 229–253. doi: 10.1057/sub.2013.9.

Stock, G. (2013). The Battle for the Future. In: M. More and N. Vita-More (Eds.): *Classical and Contemporary Essays on the Science, Technology, and Philosophy of the Human Future. The Transhumanist Reader.* Oxford: Wiley-Blackwell, 302–316.

Szakolczai, Á. (2009). Liminality and Experience: Structuring Transitory Situations and Transformative Events. *International Political Anthropology*, 2, 1, 141–172.

Szakolczai, Á. (2017). Permanent (Trickster) Liminality: The Reason of the Heart and of the Mind. *Theory & Psychology*, 27, 2, 231–248.

Thomassen, B. (2009). The Uses and Meanings of Liminality. *International Political Anthropology*, 2, 1, 5–27.

"Transhumanist Declaration (2012)" (2013). In: M. More and N. Vita-More (Eds.): *Classical and Contemporary Essays on the Science, Technology, and Philosophy of the Human Future. The Transhumanist Reader*. Oxford: Wiley-Blackwell, 54–55.

Turner, V. W. (1964). Betwixt and Between: The Liminal Period in Rites de Passage. In: J. Helm (Ed.): *Proceedings of the 1964 Annual Meeting of the American Ethnological Society: Symposium on New Approaches to the Study of Religion*. Seattle: The University of Washington Press, 4–20.

Van Gennep, A. (1960) [1909]. *The Rites of Passage*. Chicago: Chicago University Press.

Vinge, V. (2013). Technological Singularity. In: M. More and N. Vita-More (Eds.): *Classical and Contemporary Essays on the Science, Technology, and Philosophy of the Human Future. The Transhumanist Reader*. Oxford: Wiley-Blackwell, 365–375.

Chapter 2

Prolegomena to any ethical reflection on enhancement

Josef Kuře

Abstract: The chapter provides a proposal for procedural framework of any meaningful ethical reflection on human enhancement, mapping the individual steps of such a reflection. If we want to start an efficient discourse on enhancement, we first need to have a clear ontology of enhancement (what enhancement is) and have clarity about the basic semantics of enhancement, i.e. in which sense and in which lexicological extent the term "enhancement" is being used. Are all types of enhancement (such as physical, mood, cognitive, and age enhancement) included? Or are only some types included? Or do we solely refer to one type? Furthermore, it is necessary to specify the relation of the concept of enhancement to therapy (medical paradigm), and similarly we must also specify the level of enhancement (cellular, organic, implants, genomic, etc.). Enhancement challenges our understanding of medicine as well as the goals of medicine (transformative paradigm). Age enhancement is used as an example for the procedural framework of ethics while raising philosophical, psychological, social, and political questions. First, we need to understand the biology of aging. We also need to investigate issues like the life cycle, the psychology of aging, personal identity, etc. on an individual and existential level. Also, it is necessary study the consequences of aging on a social level (family, relationships, demography, population, social cohesion, etc.). Social-economic and healthcare-economic consequences also have to be analysed. Moreover our understanding of human beings, society, and the future needs to be clarified. Only then we can ask the ethical question if human enhancement can be considered good or bad, right or wrong, including normative and regulative aspects of the social and ethical acceptance of enhancement.

Introduction[1]

The phenomenon called enhancement, although it is often discussed as a single item, represents a greatly differentiated, extensive, and multilevel issue. It is where the age-old human desire for growth, progress and improvement of life conditions meet with the new technical possibilities. This desire is met with the historically unprecedented development of biomedicine which has been made possible by the enormous progress in science and biotechnologies. The idea of transgressing natural givens and

[1] The text is a modified part of the chapter Kuře, J. (2015) „Enhancement: Konceptuální ujasnění a základní podoby [Enhancement: A conceptual clarification and the basic forms of enhancement].

improving is not new, but is as old as humankind itself (Passmore 2000). Transgressing these givens, as well as surpassing what has already been achieved by an individual and society, together belongs to the foundations of human life. Carrying out life as a way of transcendence of the given has been considerably intensified and accelerated by technology. This effort to transgress the given has dramatically changed from the past thanks to radically new technological procedures that are currently available, including those that expand the options of support and the development of human health. This extensive growth of technology and biomedicine have become a fascination which could lead to the fulfilling of some of the age-old human wishes such as achieving "eternal youth" (or at least longevity) and dramatically upgrading all human abilities (Lüthy 2013).

1. Ontology and semantics

Enhancement as the use of technology implies a number of ethical and social questions (Blank 2016, Bostrom 2014, Budinger et al. 2000, Buchanan 2011, Cabrera 2015, Caplan 2006, Fuchs 2002, Lilley 2013, McKenny 2000, Parens 1998a, Savulescu 2009). The ethical questions of enhancement are preceded by the ontological question: What in fact is enhancement? One of the essential conceptual issues is the connection between enhancement and therapy. That is why some authors suggest that the term "enhancement" should only be used for non-therapeutic procedures and that it only be reserved for the use of some specific genetic and cybernetic technologies, neurotechnologies, nanotechnologies, etc. in biomedicine, so that the concept of enhancement would clearly be separated from the concept of therapy. Other authors avoid differentiating between the therapeutic and non-therapeutic use of technologies, and within the broad definition of health (health in general perceived as well-being) understand enhancement conceptually as something which improves the well-being and therefore is a part of health, because it strengthens health, provides prevention and therapy of disease. In this concept, enhancement is an integral part of well-being, development, and human welfare; it is also an expression of free choice, where the individual decides about themselves based on their personal preferences and takes responsibility for their own health and life. In this case, enhancement fits the individualistic concept of medicine as providing services which an individual demands based on their own preferences. In the concept, enhancement is also an expression of socially-ethical responsibility to public health, the development and support of the population's health, and healthcare on an all-society level. Enhancement as the support of health then becomes a social imperative in public health, and the health of the population and the government should strongly support enhancement as a form of care for the population's health. In this concept, both on an individual and social-population scale, healthy individuals should also be provided with medical services that are beyond the traditional goals of medicine. So far, the objective of medicine was to strengthen health, prevent illness, and cure disease. Until now, the therapeutic maximum of medicine has been to improve a pathological decline caused by certain illnesses to its physiological norm. Medicine has not dealt with ways to upgrade the physiological norm to a hyperphysiological level (Luber & Lisanby, 2014). Exactly this upgrade from a physiological to a hyperphysiological level is the idea of enhancement. Enhancement could also be - in case of its integration into the concept of therapy - the elevation from a physiological decline to a physiological norm.

Others, rather than the option of "improvement" ("amelioration") - which is the term used when translating enhancement into many languages, unless they choose to use the term "enhancement" as *terminus technicus*[2] - prefer eugenics as an early selection based on genome (Agar 2005; Savulescu 2001, 2006).[3] With a certain simplification, enhancement is a situation when biotechnologies can be used to help people think better, look better, feel happier, live a longer and better life, and improve their perfor-

---

[2] For example, in German, besides the English term (Enhancement), the term "Verbesserung" (improvement, improving), "Verbesserung des Menschen" (improving humans) is used. It is similar in other Germanic languages, where the English term "enhancement" is translated as "improvement": "verbetering" in Dutch ("menselijke verbetering" - human enhancement), "förbättring" in Swedish, "forbedring" in Norwegian. The same logic of translation, derived from the Latin comparative "melior" (better), appears in Romance languages: "amélioration" in French ("amélioration humaine" - human improvement/amelioration/enhancement), "miglioramento" in Italian ("miglioramento umano"), "mejoramiento" in Spanish. Elsewhere, the translation of the English term "enhancement" as "improvement in quality" divert from "improvement" towards "increasing" or "expanding", which relates to a different English term, that is "augmentation" (increase, growth, expansion) and the related term "empowerment" as possible synonyms for enhancement. For example, in Italian in this context we can find terms like "aumento", "accrescimento", "rinforzo", "potenziamento umano", in French "augmentation" and "renforcement", in Spanish "aumento" and "acrecentamiento". An interesting lexicological oscillation is visible in Polish, where the equivalent for "enhancement" is "zwiększenie", "uwydatnienie" (augmentation), "wzmocnienie" (empowerment) and "udoskonalanie (człowieka)" (making human better/perfect).

[3] One of the main critics of liberal eugenics is Jürgen Habermas (*Die Zukunft der menschlichen Natur. Auf dem Wege zu einer liberalen Eugenik?* Frankfurt am Main: Suhrkamp, 2001).

mance. An important criteria is the imperative: not just "good" but "better", not just "happy" but "happier". The comparative in this case exceeds the positive of commonality, standard, "normal" (Miller & Wilsdon, 2006). The expected "improvement" ("amelioration") is based on the "normal" use of biomedical technologies, as they are used in therapeutic procedures when an illness is treated and suffering is eased or removed. The therapeutic effectiveness of these technologies secondarily becomes a means of improving feelings, experiencing, intellectual or physical performance.

For the clarification of what enhancement is, what it is based on, and what are its targets, it is important to differentiate between medical procedures (therapy) and procedures which are beyond medical professionalism (enhancement). "One approach to the enhancement/treatment distinction is to define it in terms of the accepted limits of professional medical practice. Under this view, treatments are any interventions that physicians and their patients agree are useful and proper, while enhancements are simply interventions that are considered to fall beyond a physician's professional purview. [...] This view resonates well with a number of contemporary social-scientific critiques of biomedicine, which suggest that medicine has no natural domain of practice beyond that, which it negotiates with society." (Parens 2004, 753) Differentiating between enhancement and therapy not only allows us to set the limits between health and illness, but is also important for setting the moral implications of therapy and enhancement (McKenny 2000, Resnik 2000, Lenk 2002, Wolpe 2003, Gert & Culver 2005).

For establishing the term "enhancement" it is important to clarify how it is connected to the concept of therapy, because this clarification of terms immediately affects the ethical assessment of enhancement. While therapy has a higher moral status in the sense of moral obligation and urgency or possibly as a moral therapeutic imperative, enhancement, if it is not a part of therapy at the same time, is more a matter of personal preferences and therefore has a different moral status than therapy. But differentiating between what is therapy and what is enhancement is very difficult (Bostrom & Roache 2014, 227): "Some argue that medicine's lacks of an essential domain of practice means that a coherent distinction between medical and nonmedical services can never be drawn in the first place. [...] ...for psychological and economical reasons, a professional medical line between treatment and enhancement will be impossible to maintain in practice." (Parens 2004, 753) This distinction is often practically impossible and at the same time very important if we are to accept the semantic identity of the terms "therapy" and "enhancement", where "enhancement" contains two segments: therapy and individual preferences (Daniels 2000, Schwartz 2005).

Eric Parens (2004, 753–755) suggests the use of the three following criteria for clearly differentiating between therapy and enhancement:

a) If the given procedure is part of the medical profession (Professional Domain Approach);
b) If it is a part of normal or necessary healthcare or luxury services (Normalcy Approach);
c) If it is a solution to the consequences of illness (treatment) or enhancement as the support of health and normal characteristics (Disease-Based Approach).

Interpretations which compare therapy opposed to enhancement are especially useful in cases that set the limits of medical practice. It doesn't matter if the definition of medicine is determined by the concept of disease, the sociology of the medical profession, or the normative theory; this definition offers a tool for setting the limits, which are not limits of medical tolerance but of medical obligation (Parens 2004, 756).

The difficulty of differentiating between therapy and enhancement can be illustrated on the example of the use of the Human Growth Hormone (HGH) (Tauer 2000, Conrad & Potter 2004); a single technology (chemical substance) can both represent therapy and enhancement. It is a therapy in the case of congenital insufficiency of the HGH; in this case the application of artificially prepared HGH causes the individual to reach normal height and therefore remove their psychological and social disadvantage (Kranzler et al. 1999, Bolt et al. 2001, Voss 2001). It will not be enhancement. On the other hand, in the case of an individual with normal height (without any hormonal dysfunction), HGH will be applied to achieve a taller (than normal) figure (e.g. to be able to become a basketball player); it will be enhancement.[4] In this case, it is obvious that the usage is not therapeutic and we are beyond the limits of medicine or at least medicine as we currently understand it - that is a means of preventing illness, providing diagnosis, and treatment of illness (Konner 1999). Cole-Turner (1998, 160) argues that it is necessary to carefully distinguish in the application of the same method to different individuals: "The same technology applied to different persons with different capabilities will in fact have similar but significantly different effects, and we must learn to understand as fully as possible the differences between persons and between the ways in which the same technology might affect them." That means it is simply not possible to say if using HGH is or is not enhancement. Critical will be the context and specific situation in which the HGH will be used as well as the target of the application (Fuchs 2002).

[4] The whole issue would be much more problematic if HGH were to be given to children.

It can only be agreed that from the point of view of healthcare, improving the quality of life,[5] strengthening the health of individuals and public health as well is a desirable change. Improving the quality of life, either biologically or psychologically, is also improving the situation of the individual and their health. A specific form of the concept of enhancement is the enhancement concerning children. This form of enhancement includes the problematic "improvement" by using prenatal selection (Saluvescu 2001, Damovsky 2001, Mauron 2015).

If as a default definition we choose the one given by the World Health Organization (WHO) since 1946 – "health is a state of complete physical, mental and social well-being and not merely the absence of disease or infirmity" – then this definition supports a large medicalization of normal human conditions.[6] Who use the broad definition of health as given by, e.g. WHO assign enhancement to healthcare. Because it is not possible to exactly differ between therapy and enhancement, every non-medical issue such as aging or shyness – within the broad concept of health suggested by "welfarists"[7] – should be solved medically. Then enhancement would be every change in the biological or psychological constitution of the individual which improves the possibility to lead a good life in the new situation that will occur thanks to this "improvement". And it is necessary not only to welcome such a possibility but to also fulfill it. We must then solve the medical application of enhancement as a social question. But we will come across the basic question which is, if everything that is technically and technologically possible, is *ipso facto* ethically right (Plotz 2003). If every technically possible "improvement" of the human condition produced by biotechnologies is good and desirable – both in the individual and social sense.

Because enhancement represents a very broad and differentiated phenomenon, just the definition of the term "enhancement" suggests an ethical assessment. The definition enhancement itself already contains another agenda, ideological presumptions or postulates and therefore a given moral evaluation without declaring this agenda, ideology, or a prior evaluation beforehand. Enhancement can be defined neutrally as the use of genetic, biotechnological, or pharmaceutical knowledge to improve general

[5] Enhancement does not only mean a qualitative increase (improvement of the quality of life), but also a quantitative increase in case of prolonging life or in the previously mentioned case of applying HGH (the quantitative increase of height).
[6] According to this idealistic definition, healthy people almost do not exist. However, this official definition of health is still being used.
[7] This is the term used by Julian Savulescu (2006).

human or individual characteristics; or it can also be identified as a radical improvement *of the quality of life* using biotechnologies; or it can be described as *helping* to live a longer and better life than normally; as well as it can be identified as biotechnological *manipulation*, the *improvement of social* status, a social *deception* (Parens 2004, 755), technological *modification of humans*, an attempt to *control* the development of the individual and society, a form of biopower and a way of controlling others, a way of *altering* human nature, a violation of human nature or dignity, *crossing the natural limits*, crossing the limits of what is allowed and normal, or as a *subversion of humanity* (McWhorter 2009, Buchanan 2011b, Frippiat 2011, Goffi 2011). So not only the relation to the concept of therapy, but also depending on in which terminological and emotional context the term "enhancement" is used in will determine its ethical evaluation (e.g. improvement, modification, manipulation, subversion).

The term "enhancement" contains the moral ambivalence which reaches from "improvement" to "the subversion of humanity". If enhancement is replaced in certain languages with the semantics of "improvement" (e.g. "Verbesserung" in German, "amélioration" in French, "majoramiento" in Spanish), the moral ambivalence of enhancement is erased: Verbesserung, amelioration, or mejoramiento cannot be morally disputable or problematic, they are by definition something good because - semantically - they are derived from the comparative of "good - better".

As for extent, enhancement is a very broad phenomenon; its extent reaches from "improving" on a genomic level, through pharmaceutical "improvement" of emotions and physical possibilities of the human organism and the physical appearance, all the way to the cognitive functions and memory (Gerlai 2003, Glannon 2006) and connecting the human brain to a computer, surpassing the limits of human intelligence with artificial intelligence and reaching a state of singularity (Kurzweil 2005).

We can divide enhancement in a basic way into physical, psychological, cognitive, and age enhancement. Genetic enhancement is a specific category (Smith 2000, Bostrom 2003, Mehlman 2003, Baylis & Robert 2004, DeGrazia 2016), which modifies a gene or genes, where this genetic modification can manifest in any of the previously mentioned four areas. It is very difficult to terminologically express enhancement because of its poly-semantics and moral ambivalence. The term "enhancement" also describes a number of various procedures on a genomic, cellular, pharmacological, or physical level, in the area of communication and information technologies (implanted chips, brain-computer interface), in the area of physical appearance and performance, intellectual abilities, psychological perception, and social behavior. Just the categorization of enhancement itself illustrates the differences in approach. Besides the four mentioned categories, there are also other types of division. For example, Shapiro and his colleagues divide enhancement into "cognitive, emotional, and behavioral performance" (Shapiro et al. 2003, 1427). It is necessary to point out that genomic enhancement is from today's point of view the most futuristic version of enhancement. Unlike the modification of physical appearance or emotions, genomic enhancement is something which is not quite possible yet. But, if genomic enhancement became technically possible, it would be completely revolutionary not only for medicine.

After this brief outline of the differentiation, extent a multi-level character of the phenomenon called enhancement, it is obvious that questions such as "Are you for or against enhancement?" are incorrectly asked questions. It is impossible to simply or clearly answer these questions; or rather any answers given to such questions do not actually tell us anything. They do not inform us what the given individual thinks about enhancement as a concept and if they agree or disagree with enhancement, or with which forms they agree or disagree. It is not sufficient to just ask the questions about the moral agreement or disagreement with enhancement, but in the first place it is necessary to clarify the question of what is enhancement, so it is obvious with which resource the respondent is agreeing or disagreeing, what the debate is even about. But it is not just about clarifying the ontology of enhancement. The following part of the chapter will try to outline the circumstances for the structure of the ethical reflection of enhancement and clarify the requirements for such a discussion.[8]

2. Prior to any ethical reflection on enhancement

2.1. Enhancement as a concept and category

Before we even get into the systematic ethics of enhancement, it is necessary to specify what had to be taken into account in relation to this and clarify the requirements of the systematic reflection of enhancement. Only a very superficial observer may think that it is just a question of saying yes

[8] The necessity of clarifying these preconditions is reflected in the attempt of a systematic reflection of enhancement recently published by Allan Buchanan (2011a, 1–34).

or no to enhancement. It is not at all about this question, that is, primarily it is not about this question. Besides that, the issue of enhancement cannot simply be solved with a binary system: 1 and 0. Because some attempts of solving enhancement closely resemble exactly this approach of 1 and 0. First of all, it is a far more important question, than if simply to say yes or no to enhancement, to allow it or ban it, to regulate it and if so then how. It is possible to answer the question "Should we say yes or no to enhancement?" only after we answer some much more important questions. Generally speaking, it depends on the whole context of this discussion, its requirements, and starting point. In the end, even if a global consensus of the prohibition of enhancement was reached – though such a thing is complete fiction given the broad and deep dissent concerning enhancement as a concept and the pluralism of its ethical evaluation – it would not be wise to even wish for such a global consensus of prohibition, even if it were just as a part of an intellectual exercise. Not only would it be a regression before "scienza nuova", that is before renaissance, and also that scientific and technical development is unstoppable, there remains the question, if such a prohibition could offer any solution. Besides the conceptual understanding of enhancement, which does not separate it from therapy, would not allow such a prohibition. Enhancement as the idea of improving humans, developing their possibilities and capacities, is unstoppable, because it corresponds with the basic self-understanding of people as the ones who decide about their development and future (Baylis & Robert, 2004). But it is necessary to accompany this development with ethical reflection, to point out the connections and possible consequences – and not only the negative ones.

While discussing enhancement, it often happens that the discourse begins at the ending and the question which is dominant right from the beginning is regulation, how to regulate enhancement, which regulation tools to choose (soft law – hard law), on which levels to regulate, and how to regulate. Whereas the more fundamental question is not how or with which tools to regulate, but if to regulate at all and why we should regulate in the first place. In some discourses, enhancement ethics are replaced by enhancement governance. But in fact, enhancement governance does not replace enhancement ethics, but presumes them.

No matter how difficult it may be to exactly and clearly define enhancement, it is obvious that enhancement represents a philosophically-ethical and philosophically-anthropological challenge (Parens, 2009). The first basic obstacle is the terminological and conceptual clarification. In this sense the phenomenon enhancement – not intentionally and programmatically

– fits the concept of postmodernity and its uncertainty, ambiguity, inconsistency, and episodicity. We simply do not have a clear consensus concerning the term enhancement. Enhancement is shattered into a number of forms of improving humans, some of which have been mentioned previously. Also the poly-semantics of enhancement, without directly attempting to do so, correspond with postmodern ambiguity. On one hand, enhancement is the term for a time continuum of the efforts of humans to grow, as they have manifested in different periods in history, and on the other hand it is the discontinuity and episodicity of the life of an individual, who lives their own little personal stories, and phrasing these stories could express, in a random way, enhancement as the transition from one to another, where this transition from one to another could be understood as an augmentation of the possibilities of life.

If we ask the question whether enhancement is or is not therapy, we do not get a satisfactory answer, because we do not have clear criteria for differentiating between therapy and enhancement. If, for example, we use the definition given by WHO, then separating enhancement from therapy is practically impossible. Those, who try to assign enhancement to therapy often describe it as "substitution therapy" – but that does usually not replace a damaged function. From this point of view it would at least be a term of a not indicated therapy. Those, who do not assign enhancement to therapy, differentiate between curative and transformative procedures. From this point of view enhancement belongs to transformative procedures (Shapiro et al. 2003, 23; Agar & McDonald 2017). Due to the fact, that a single technology could be therapy in one case and an "improvement" in another, we have no other option than to strictly apply contextualization and evaluate the use of technologies from case to case while taking into account all the circumstances, conditions, and the given situation.

A part of the conceptual understanding of enhancement is semantics, which in many languages is based on "improvement" as previously mentioned (Note 2). The poly-semantics of enhancement are based on the fact that there is no single enhancement, but there are many types of enhancement and many levels on which enhancement is carried out. Enhancement can relate to many levels: gene enhancement, cellular, organic, pharmaceutical, etc. For clarifying the type of enhancement, the basic requirement is understanding, i.e, the correct understanding of the biological and physiological foundations of enhancement; this means an undistorted understanding of the factual side of enhancement.

The phenomenon enhancement non-thematically suggests which themes are even part of prospective thinking, a type of thinking that is concentrated on the future, the future as such - that means not just the future that would be - in the sense of Jonas's ontology of the responsibility for humans, that is for humans to exist and therefore a future to exist (Jonas 1984, 79–94 and 184–187) - but more importantly how the future will be, what will society be like in the future, what will the basic conception of a person be in the future society both on a social and individual level (the concept of personal identity, authenticity, etc.).

Further will be indicated all that is at play in reflecting these biomedical technologies and what the possibilities which we call "human enhancement" concern and which questions and issues implicitly lay behind these strictly technological possibilities. To outline the elements of ethical reflection, not all types and levels of enhancement will be taken into account, but for clarity we will use just a single case and that is age enhancement. On the case of age enhancement, we will be exemplifying the conditions and structure of the reflection of enhancement.[9] Enhancement is a very differentiated phenomenon. That is why it is not possible to ethically reflect it as a single element, if this evaluation should not end up in the previously mentioned polarity of the binary system (1 and 0). A number of conditions which are mentioned (e.g. the clarification of terms, the idea of future society, and the place of an individual in it) are applicable to all types of enhancement, and some are specific for age enhancement.

2.2. Age enhancement as an example of structural conditions for the ethical reflection of enhancement

Prolonging human age is a very old idea (Gruman 2003). But for centuries its realization was impossible due to the lack of effective "life elixirs", which in the future are to be represented by biotechnology: "We see the prospect of further increases of life span as a realistic possibility, but our ancestors were never in any doubt that ageing was inevitable and unavoidable." (Sargent 2005, 151). Age enhancement - unlike physical, cognitive, or psychological enhancement - has not gotten very far with practical applications. Actual experimental results, which we have about age enhancement, in a short period of time rather lead to certain modesty than ambitions of drastically slowing the process of aging of the organism or even stopping it and achieving immortality (Jonas 1992, Callahan 1993). But it

[9] The literature mentioned is for practical reasons of an illustrative, not an exhaustive character.

is necessary to mention that there are other areas of enhancement (e.g. cognitive or mood enhancement) where the results are more ambitious and promising.

2.2.1. Age enhancement: concept and models

Unlike other types of enhancement, it is a lot simpler to terminologically grasp age enhancement. It is the prolonging of life, a variously intensive and radical prolonging of life to the utter limit of completely stopping the biological process of aging of an organism. Besides this, what has already been stated about enhancement also applies for the term age enhancement and its terminological definition in relation to therapy.

There are many concepts concerning the possibility of prolonging life, which can be divided into the following three types of age enhancement (Juengst 2004a), which at the same time express different levels of progressivism or rather conservatism relating to prolonging the human life:

a) Compressed morbidity

The most conservative approach to the issue of prolonging life is a model called "compressed morbidity" (Fries 1988). Its main goal is to lower morbidity and prevent chronic geriatric diseases so that people are able to live longer and healthier – within the limitations of age that humans live as a biological species. This approach emphasizes the prevention of illness which is connected to old age; its aim is to lengthen life expectancy and lower morbidity, but not to achieve the longest age possible. The result of this approach is a society with many elderly citizens, but who play an active part in this society until their death.

b) Decelerated aging

The goal of this approach is to slow down the process of aging as much as possible and lengthen life expectancy and maximum lifespan (Glannon 2002a, Harris & Holm 2002, Kogan et al. 2011). If the process of aging is slowed down, people could normally live to be 100 years old, more optimistic estimations suggest even 140 years old (Miller 2002). But the question is to what age would people be relatively healthy and how would morbidity express in a longer age. The common belief of this group of gerontologists is the hypothesis that we would enjoy good health even in high age.

c) Negligible senescence

This model takes into account the possibility of a gradual avert of the process of aging, which normally occurs in all adult individuals (Fossel 1996). The goal of this form of enhancement is to keep unlimited vitality and remove old age as a problem (Grey 2007). A way of achieving this goal could be to remove defects that occur during metabolic processes which would lead to the unlimited postponing of aging; humans would be redesigned in their time-space existence (Stock 2002). This model is based on the assumption that "managing" the process of aging (in the sense of continual postponing of aging) will be possible in the first half of the 21st century (Grey et al. 2002, Hayflick 2007). Aging, which in this concept is something negligible, responds to the pursuit of surpassing the limitations of medicine and human existence: the barrier of death will be overcome and the possibilities of permanent existence will open up, that is immortality (Olshansky & Carnes 2001, Zaleski 2004, Miller & Wilsdon 2006).

The three different concepts of prolonging life reflect in various ways into the concept of human enhancement as a form of prolonging human life. Prolonging life then indirectly suggests that "longer" is "better". Whereas in the first case, (compressed) morbidity is a preventive model, where the principle of enhancement is to prevent illnesses which are typical for old age - and such a model can medically and ethically only be welcomed - the second model (decelerated aging), which means the slowing of the process of aging, needs differentiating - e.g. in relation to how this slowing of aging would be achieved. Is it deceleration as a result of a healthy lifestyle or of a biotechnological intervention? If a person leads a healthy life, avoids smoking, stress, unhealthy meals and overeating, lives in harmony in their relationships and existential comfort, it is without doubt an "improvement" of life compared to those who do not live healthily - it is therefore enhancement in its broadest sense. The instance the length of human life is prolonged by some of the biotechnological methods, it brings up a number of individual ethical and socially ethical questions. The third model (negligible senescence), which is a complete negation of aging and old age, is a radical model and ethically and socially the most problematic. The question remains whether surpassing the limits of mortality - however it may correspond with cultural archetypes of "eternal youth" and the historical efforts of humans to achieve time and space of immortality (McGee 2007) - is a part of science fiction rather than a solid intellectual or scientific project.

Just the presentation of these three basic models of age enhancement clearly shows that the question whether to say yes or no to enhancement is incorrectly placed, and there is no correct answer to it and either versions of the answer does not tell us much.

2.2.2. Preliminary results in age enhancement

An area in which we have certain, mostly experimental, results is the research of reducing the amount of calories given to some model species of animals (Sohal & Weindruch, 1996, Rebrin et al. 2011, Wegman et al. 2015). The question remains, if this method of calorie restriction is applicable to humans, because it is connected to side effects such as psychological stress, hunger, lower physical performance, etc.

Another area is the research of the HGH. It has turned out that when given to older individuals it strengthens the immune system, causes growth of muscle, and lowers body fat (Blackman et al. 2002, Nass 2013). But the use of Growth Hormone on animal subjects has shown serious side effects, especially a higher occurrence of cancer, diabetes, and hypertension (Hintz 2004). This shows that the use of HGH as enhancement is currently clinically impossible.

The genetic modification of Embryonic Stem Cells (ESCs) would also belong into this group and further the production of immunologically compatible tissues or organs in laboratory circumstances for the purpose of transplantation enhancement or for the purpose of influencing the process of cellular aging (Hertzog 2006, Rodriguez-Brenes & Peskin 2010, He et al. 2014, Zou et al. 2017). From the point of view of our current knowledge of the process of cellular differentiation and our still very limited abilities to control this process, this form of prolonging age (simply for the reason of safety of such modifications) is at the moment only a theory - which does not exclude that it may be a real possibility in the future (Overall 2009). Aging is a biological, psychological, and social process and recently a closely monitored theme (Callahan 1987, Daniels 1988, Kirkwood 1999, Overall 2003, Olshansky 2016, Roduit 2016).

2.2.3. Age enhancement and time

It is obvious that medicine of the 20th century has significantly contributed to the prolonging of human life. But most likely we will not call this documented prolongation *enhancement*. If medicine of the first half of the 20th century and the first decades of the 21st century has set its goal to postpone death, or more precisely scientific and technological development has assigned it this goal and medicine has quietly accepted it, then shouldn't this task be taken on with new vehemence in the area of age enhancement and shouldn't we try even harder to postpone the issue of death? Or, as some in medicine suggest, solve the issue of mortality once and for all? This is obviously connected to the limitation of medicine and redefining the goals of medicine (Juengst 2004b, 321–339). The question is whether medicine should only solve pathologies and with its preventive and therapeutic procedures add to the quality of human life or if it should also add length to human life, eventually both. It is good to remind that medicine has, by eradicating infectious diseases of the 20th century, objectively added this time. On the other hand, it is also true that vaccination, which was and still is a medical tool of prevention and of prolonging human life on a population level, is not in any context indicated as human enhancement (Binstock 2004, 11–37).

Age *enhancement*, especially in its radical form (negligible senescence), is an attempt to surpass the limits of human existence in time and space (Agar 2014). Though it is not very likely that the research of the process of aging and "anti-aging medicine" (Juengst et al. 2003, de Gray 2004, Holstein et al. 2011, 87–102) will be able to provide genetic alteration of the process of aging or its complete stopping any time soon, nevertheless age enhancement represents an impulse, leading us to a number of questions.

2.2.4. Not solely technical issues

If the prolonging of life were to happen on a cellular level, then the first questions would be the matter of safety of such a procedure (Kamm 2005) and the issue of risk – so that the results would be prolonging and not shortening life or prolonging life but with a lower quality. Even provided, though from the perspective of today's knowledge in the field of cellular biology only hypothetically, that the process of cellular intervention would be a completely safe procedure without any risk (e.g. cancer transformations), the spread of these technologies would have serious social consequences (Chapman 2004).

The first and most obvious consequence would be an increase in population size on a global scale. This event would – without taking into account the current population explosion – bring a number of unfortunate consequences, such as issues with the quality of life or fights for basic resources such as drinking water, food, medical care, which would at the same time become rare resources, or rather even more rare. Liberal democratic states would then be under the temptation to authoritatively intervene into reproduction rights, less developed democracies would probably not be able to withstand such a growth in population and would apply very drastic population and other social legislative measurements. To create and apply corresponding politics of long age on a global scale would be very difficult for very serious implications, which radically prolonging life would bring. The implication of longevity on a local scale would bring other types of issues between societies with longevity and those without it, as well as within the societies with longevity themselves.

2.2.5. Access to age enhancement

Even with the otherwise legitimate precondition, which is the concept of a neutral liberal state, that does not interfere with biology or psychology and reserves it for individuals to decide within their own freedom and autonomy based on their personal preferences and various concepts of "good life" and does not leave these decisions even to "experts" (biologists, philosophers, sociologists, psychologists) or "nature", or not to secular or religious authorities (state, government, doctors, churches), the basic question remains, if age enhancement would be financed on a personal-individual basis of this liberal precondition and the matter of enhancement would be regulated by free market economy, or if the state would provide equal access to these technologies within the state guaranteed healthcare and if enhancement would belong to the right for healthcare and therefore to the basic rights of every citizen of European democracies. Just like patients today have the right to healthcare in countries with public healthcare, these patients suffering from the illness called old age would have the right to longevity,[10] especially if age enhancement was considered a part of therapy.

Because the result of the process of slowing aging or "removing" old age would also be a significant disproportional change in the ratio between old and young people in favor of the older ones, a general result of this enhancement would be jeopardizing the intergenerational equity – there would be less and less of economically active (younger) people, opposed to that the percentage of economically inactive (older) people which would gradually be growing, i.e, percentage of those which would need an increasing amount of funds for providing basic needs and health and social care. This disproportional model of allocated resources is in contrast with the model in which funds from health insurance are divided to allow all individuals to live a normal life expectancy, and those who cross this limit are not denied healthcare but are in a certain way reduced (Callahan 1987, Daniels 1988). The statement, that age is not an indicating

[10] Though old age is not considered an illness nowadays, there are a number of illnesses which in the past were also not considered to be an illness.

criteria even in recent healthcare, remains in many cases a mere proclamation. The criteria of age is already being applied in common clinical practice nowadays, when it comes to the allocation and distribution of rare resources (e.g. transplantations or financially very demanding treatments).

If we take into account the growing disproportion between technical possibilities of biomedicine and the growing but nevertheless principally limited funds for providing healthcare in many countries, we find ourselves at the basic issue of the concept of medicine. If we decide to support the model of "sustainable medicine" (Callahan 1999, 25–45 and 240–289), which is affordable in the long run, then it is obvious that it will not be possible to finance some procedures from the funds of health insurance and that a significant prolonging of life, which is not a pathology or a dysfunction – assuming that old age and aging are not a disease or pathology – will not be assigned as a model of sustainable medicine.

2.2.6. The quest for normalcy

It is quite difficult to conceptually determine what the "normal" length of life actually is. It used to be half as long as today not so many years ago, and even today it is nearly half the length in a number of countries compared to the European-American civilization. The "normal" length of life is a social construct which changes according to the social consensus. It is similarly difficult to speak about prolonging the "normal" length of life. The "normal" functioning of an organism is a changing variable, which is determined socially, culturally, and geographically. What is the "normal" length of life on a global scale at the beginning of the 21st century? Is it the global average length? Would it be incorrect to globally apply this average "normal" length of life? Or will we calculate with the "normal" length of life in single societies?

In the last two centuries, average life expectancy has more than doubled and is still growing, but this only applies to developed countries (Sargent 2005, 312–314). And what about "undeveloped" parts of the world? Is it legitimate and compatible with the concept of solidarity and social cohesion, for the western world, which is consuming most of the world's resources, to develop technologies that will then only serve one part of the world and that will improve the health and prolong the "normal" life expectancy of a small percentage of the global population and in this way be creating social tension, barriers, and intergenerational problems, while a much larger portion of the inhabitants of the planet and especially the younger generations will be excluded from the current and prospective benefits of these technologies in advance and will be sentenced to a completely different "normality"? Isn't it an ethically questionable concept to prolong the age of a small portion of the world's population while a large portion of this population does not have access to basic healthcare? Said with a certain exaggeration, wouldn't the price for "achieving longevity", for "removing old age", or even "overcoming death" be social suicide?

2.2.7. Meaningfulness of aging

In the end it is not clear at all, if significant prolonging of life or even "removing old age" would be beneficial to humans (Glannon 2002b), if it isn't just playing with the idea of longevity or immortality rather than something, that we would as individuals really want, prefer, or should strive to achieve. "Whether or not the biological changes of aging are beneficial or harmful, they are meaningful: They and their natural timing constitute part of normal life cycle for human beings, and thus part of what it means to be human. Intentionally distorting that cycle alienates the elderly from the definitive human life story, and dehumanizes them in the process. In this view, adults should be taught to seek the meaning of the later stages of human development, and biomedical research should focus on making the experience of that part of life as healthy and pleasant as possible, but not interfere in its essential rhythm." (Juengst 2004a, 114) From the point of view of developmental psychology and personality psychology, aging is an important process in our human maturing, and old age is an inseparable part of our lives and our personal identity. According to Erik Erikson (1982), old age is a key moment of the life cycle.

The concept of slowing or stopping the process of aging (within the so-called anti-aging medicine) is just as fascinating, as it brings up a number of ethical, psychological, social, and political questions (Neugarten & Havighurst 1977, Selzer 1995, Miller 2002, 2006). Age enhancement is not just a matter of personal ethics, but a social ethical matter, just as it is a matter of philosophical anthropology and a matter of social or political philosophy.

2.2.8. The levels of age enhancement discourse

It is necessary to examine the issue of lifespan enhancement on a number of levels:

a) on a scientific and factual level (biology of aging);

b) on a conceptual and semantic level (which term of enhancement to use, what type and kind of enhancement is meant);
c) on the level of philosophical anthropology (what term and vision of a human we use, which content we assign to humanity, what hermeneutics of self-concept we use and how we understand self-fulfillment, if we understand humans in the humanistic sense of "Become, who you are!" or we understand them as projects which constantly needs to evolve and grow, or more radically, as something that in the Nietzschean sense or in the sense of Transhumanism must perish and be overcome as an Übermensch (Superhuman, Transhuman), how we approach the factual and principal limitation of humans in time and space);
d) on an individual existential level (life cycle, the psychological process of aging, the "normality" of aging, the meaning of aging and old age for the development of the individual, personal preferences, identity, authenticity);
e) on the level of small social units such as family (the consequences of longevity for the concept of family and family relationships, the social function and meaning of aging, and old age in the context of family and family relationships);
f) on the level of demographics (the consequences of longevity on the demographic structure of the population);
g) on a social level (the consequences of longevity on society as a whole and its functioning, what our idea is and what future we want for ourselves and the following generations);
h) on an economical level (especially health-economical and social-economical approaches to age enhancement);
i) on a political and legislative level (corresponding political and legislative decisions adjusting the field of a meaningful functioning of society while taking into account the bearing capacity of a significantly demographically changed population).

Only after a thorough discussion of the issue of "life extension" on all levels, it would be possible to state a discussion about whether with good factual knowledge and a relatively clear idea of a prospective society with a significantly demographically changed structure, we will try to achieve age enhancement, which model of age enhancement will this society try to achieve, including the models of stopping the process of aging and fulfilling the ancient old human desire for "eternal youth". Only then can we start answering the question if enhancement is good or right in a qualified way, if its realization is a good or right choice and action. So far it seems that we have a number of serious issues of a very different nature, and it is also true that the discussion about age enhancement is a matter of a limited number of those interested and remains an academic discussion from a large part. What has been previously stated about levels on which it is necessary to explore this phenomenon of "life extension", could also be said for every kind of technological "improvement" (modification, enhancement) of humans.

Conclusion

The intention of this text was to show which questions we need to ask, before this very simple question is placed: "Is enhancement right or wrong?" In other words the aim was to specify which questions this simple question involves and contains at the same time.

It has turned out that it is quite difficult to categorize enhancement and exactly differ among the individual types of enhancement. It is similarly difficult to reach a final consensus concerning enhancement as a concept and its relation to therapy, and with that also its place in medicine and healthcare. At the same time, this terminological differentiation is a necessary predisposition for further ethical evaluation.

Enhancement as a phenomenon also refers to the issue of the limitation of human existence, technology, and medicine. It may seem that today's technological medicine brings unlimited, or almost unlimited, technological possibilities, which in comparison with procedures available a couple decades ago can almost do the impossible. Nevertheless, the subject of these technologies is humans, who are limited entities, in the end limited by their mortality. Just like medicine where the diagnostic and therapeutic possibilities have expanded in a great way in the last couple of decades, both science and art (iatriké téchne) have remained limited entities. Though in biomedicine the knowledge and number of individual diagnostic and therapeutic methods has been continually growing – including "improvement" methods (regardless whether the "disorder model" is used for enhancement or not) –, biomedicine remains a principally limited medicine. The limitation of medicine has three different causes, which are the limitation of human knowledge, the limitation of technology as a product of humans, and the limitation of human existence in time and space. Enhancement can also be a form of scientism, which conceals the (pseudo) religious ambition of the self-transcendence of humans.

The question is how does medicine, in a society oriented on performance and success (and western enhancement fits this model of thinking), deal with its own limitation - if it perceives it as an integral part or as an imperfection, failure and negative, that needs to be overcome. Or if enhancement, whether it is age or cognitive or psychological enhancement, is the way and possibility, how to surpass or finally overcome this crucial limitation? In every case, enhancement as a model offers a tool to overcome the current limitations of human abilities and the limitation of human existence. Is it instrumental reason that frees us from our (natural) limitations? In this sense enhancement completely fits the project of modernism and its late stage called postmodernism. The questions remains, if it is correct that "more is better" and "unlimited is best"? Is the enhanced human a way of overcoming the human condition, a path to Übermensch (as a form of radical enhancement) or to the self (Jungian "das Selbst")? Does enhancement cause a new estrangement of a person to themselves or does it bring them closer to themselves? How does enhancement correlate with our idea of society in which we would like to live in and which we would wish the future generations to live in? This is why there is no other option than to carefully differentiate and think before one model of enhancement or another is launched.

Literature

Agar, N. (2005) *Liberal Eugenics: In Defence of Human Enhancement*, Malden: Blackwell Publishing.

Agar, N. (2014) *Truly Human Enhancement: A Philosophical Defense of Limits*, Cambridge/MA: MIT Press.

Agar, N. and McDonald, J. (2017) Human enhancement and the story of Job, *Cambridge Quarterly of Healthcare Ethics* 26 (3), 449–458.

Baylis, F. and Robert, J. S. (2004) The inevitability of genetic enhancement technologies, *Bioethics* 8 (1), 1–26.

Binstock, R. H. (2004) The search for longevity: A contentious pursuit, in Post, S. G., Binstock, R. H. (Eds) *The Fountain of Youth. Cultural, Scientific, and Ethical Perspectives on Biomedical Goal*, Oxford - New York: Oxford University Press, 11–37.

Blackman, M. R., Sorkin, J. D. et al. (2002) Growth hormone and sex steroid administration in healthy aged women and men: A randomized controlled trial, *Journal of the American Medical Association (JAMA)* 288 (12), 2282–2292.

Blank, R. H. (2016) *Cognitive Enhancement: Social and Public Policy Issues*, New York: Palgrave Macmillan.

Bolt, L. E. and Mul, D. (2001) Growth hormone in short children: Beyond medicine? *Acta Paediatrica* 90 (1), 69–73.

Bostrom, N. (2003) Human genetic enhancements: A transhumanist perspective, *Journal of Value Inquiry* 37 (4), 493–506.

Bostrom, N. (2014) *Superintelligence: Paths, Dangers, Strategies*, Oxford: Oxford University Press.

Bostrom, N. and Roache, R. (2014) Ethical issues in human enhancement, in Boylan, M. (Ed) *Medical Ethics*, 2nd edition, Malden – Oxford: Willey-Blackwell, 226–251.

Buchanan, A. (2011a) *Beyond Humanity? The Ethics of Biomedical Enhancement*, Oxford – New York: Oxford University Press.

Buchanan, A. (2011b) *Better than Human: The Promise and Perils of Enhancing Ourselves*, Oxford – New York: Oxford University Press.

Budinger, T. F. et al. (2000) Human enhancement, in Murray, T. M., Mehlman, M. J. (Eds) *Encyclopedia of Ethical, Legal, and Policy Issues in Biotechnology*, New York: John Wiley & Sons, Vol. I, 485–552.

Cabrera, L.Y. (2015) *Rethinking Human Enhancement: Social Enhancement and Emergent Technologies*, New York: Palgrave Macmillan.

Callahan, D. (1987) *Setting Limits: Medical Goals in an Aging Society*, New York: Simon & Schuster.

Callahan, D. (1999) *False Hopes. Overcoming the Obstacles to a Sustainable, Affordable Medicine*, New Brunswick: Rutgers University Press.

Caplan, A. L. (2006) Is it wrong to try to improve human nature? in Miller, P., Wilsdon, J. (Eds) *Better Humans? The Politics of Human Enhancement and Life Extension*, London: Demos, 31–39.

Chapman, A. R. (2004) The social and justice implications of extending the human life span, in Post, S. G., Binstock, R. H. (Eds) *The Fountain of Youth. Cultural, Scientific, and Ethical Perspectives on Biomedical Goal*, Oxford – New York: Oxford University Press, 340–361.

Cole-Turner, R. (1998) Do means matter? in Parens, E. (Ed) *Enhancing Human Traits: Social and Ethical Implications*, Washington/DC: Georgetown University Press, 151–161.

Conrad, P. and Potter, D. (2004) Human growth hormone and the temptations of biomedical enhancement, *Sociology of Health and Illness* 26 (2), 184–215.

Damovsky, M. (2001) The case against designer babies: The politics of genetic enhancement, in Tokar, B. (Ed) *Redesigning Life? The Worldwide Challenge to Genetic Engineering*, London: Zed Books, 133–149.

Daniels, N. (1988) *Am I My Parents' Keeper? An Essay on Justice Between the Young and the Old*, New York: Oxford University Press.

Daniels, N. (2000) Normal functioning and the treatment-enhancement distinction, *Cambridge Quarterly of Healthcare Ethics* 9(3), 309–322.

DeGrazia, D. (2016) Ethical reflections on genetic enhancement with the aim of enlarging altruism, *Health Care Analysis* 24 (3), 180–195.

Erikson, E. (1982) *The Life Cycle Completed: A Review*, New York: Norton.

Fossel, M. (1996) *Reversing Human Aging*, New York: William Morrow.

Fries, J. (1988) Aging, illness, and health policy: Implications of the compression of morbidity, *Perspectives in Biology and Medicine* 31 (3), 407–428.

Frippiat, L. (2011) L'amélioration technique de l'être humain: introduction aux différents courants du débat, *Journal International de Bioéthique* 3–4 (22), 33–50.

Fuchs, M. (2002) Die Einschätzung des Kleinwuchses als ein Streitfall im Recht und die medizinethische Debatte um Therapie und Enhancement (Verbesserung), in Honnefelder, L., Streffer, C. (Eds) *Jahrbuch für Wissenschaft und Ethik*, Berlin - New York: de Gruyter, Vol. VII, 283–293.

Gerlai, R. (2003) Memory enhancement: The progress and our fears, *Genes, Brain and Behavior* 2 (4), 187–190.

Gert, B. and Culver, C. M. (2005) Therapy and enhancement, in Mitcham, C. (Ed) *Encyclopedia of Science, Technology, and Ethics*, Farmington Hills: Thomson & Gale, 1938–1942.

Glannon, W. (2002a) Extending the human life span, *Journal of Medicine and Philosophy* 27 (3), 339–354.

Glannon, W. (2002b) Identity, prudential concern, and extending lives, *Bioethics* 16 (3), 266–283.

Glannon, W. (2006) Psychopharmacology and memory, *Journal of Medical Ethics* 32 (2), 74–78.

Goffi, J.-Y. (2011) Nature humaine et amélioration de l'être humain à la lumière du programme transhumaniste, *Journal International de Bioéthique* 3–4 (22), 18–32.

Grey de, A. D. N. J. (2004) An engineer's approach to developing real anti-aging medicine, in Post, S. G., Binstock, R. H. (Eds) *The Fountain of Youth. Cultural, Scientific, and Ethical Perspectives on Biomedical Goal*, Oxford - New York: Oxford University Press, 249–270.

Grey de, A. (2007) *Ending Aging: The Rejuvenation Breakthroughs That Could Reverse Human Aging in Our Lifetime*, New York: St. Martin's Press.

Grey de, A., Ames, B. N., Andersen, J. K. (2002) Time to talk SENS: Critiquing the immutability of human aging, *Annals of the New York Academy of Sciences* 959, 452–462.

Gruman, G. J. (2003) *A History of Ideas About the Prolongation of Life*, New York: Springer.

Habermas, J. (2001) *Die Zukunft der menschlichen Natur. Auf dem Wege zu einer liberalen Eugenik?* Frankfurt am Main: Suhrkamp.

Harris, J. (1999) Is gene therapy a form of eugenics? in Kuhse, H., Singer, P. (Eds) *Bioethics. An Anthology*, Oxford: Blackwell, 165–170.

Harris, J., Holm, S. (2002) Extending human lifespan and the precautionary paradox, *Journal of Medicine and Philosophy* 27 (3), 355–368.

Hayflick, L. (2007) Biological aging is no longer an unsolved problem, *Annals of the New York Academy of Sciences* 1100, 1–13.

He, L., Zheng, Y., Wan, Y., Song, J. (2014) A shorter telomere is the key factor in preventing cultured human mesenchymal stem cells from senescence escape, *Histochemistry and Cell Biology* 142 (3), 257–267.

Hertzog, R.G. (2006) Ancestral telomere shortening: A countdown that will increase mean life span? *Medical Hypothesis* 67 (1), 157–160.

Hintz, R. L. (2004) Growth hormone: Uses and abuses, *British Medical Journal* 328 (7445), 907–908.

Holstein, M. B., Parks, J. A., Waymack, M. H. (2011) *Ethics, Aging, and Society: The Critical Turn*, New York: Springer.

Jonas, H. (1984) *Das Prinzip Verantwortung: Versuch einer Ethik für die technologische Zivilisation*, Frankfurt am Main: Suhrkamp.

Jonas, H. (1992) The burden and blessing of mortality, *Hastings Center Report* 22 (1), 34–40.

Juengst, E. T. (2004a) Anti-aging interventions: Ethical and social issues, in Post, S. G. (Ed) *Encyclopedia of Bioethics*, 3rd edition, New York – Detroit: Thomson, Macmillan Reference, Vol. I, 112–116.

Juengst, E. T. (2004b) Anti-aging medicine and the limits of medicine, in Post, S. G., Binstock, R. H. (Eds) *The Fountain of Youth. Cultural, Scientific, and Ethical Perspectives on Biomedical Goal*, Oxford – New York: Oxford University Press, 321–338.

Juengst, E. T., Binstock, R. H., Mehlman, M. J., Post, S. G, Whitehouse, P. (2003) Biogerontology, "anti-aging medicine", and the challenges of human enhancement, *Hastings Center Report* 33 (4), 21–30.

Kamm, F. M. (2005) Is there a problem with enhancement, *American Journal of Bioethics* 5 (3), 5–14.

Kirkwood, T. (1999) *Time of Our Lives: The Science of Human Aging*, New York: Oxford University Press.

Kogan, N., Tucker, J., Porter, M. (2011) Extending the human life span: An exploratory study of pro- and anti-longevity attitudes, *International Journal of Aging and Human Development* 73 (1), 1–25.

Konner, M. J. (1999) One pill makes you larger. The ethics of enhancement, *Minnesota Medicine* 82 (8), 26–32.

Kranzler, J. H., Rosenbloom, A. L., Proctor, B., Diamond, F. B., Watson, M. (1999) Is short stature a handicap? A comparison of the psychosocial functioning of referred and nonreffered children with normal short stature and children with normal stature, *Journal of Pediatrics* 136 (1), 96–102.

Kuře, J. (2015) Enhancement: Konceptuální ujasnění a základní podoby, in Payne, J., Černý, D., Doležal, A. et al. *Dobrý nebo lepší život? Human Enhancement*, Praha: Ústav státu a práva AV ČR, 13–43.

Kurzweil, R. (2005) *The Singularity Is Near: When Humans Transcend Biology*, New York: Viking.

Lenk, C. (2002) *Therapie und Enhancement: Ziele und Grenzen der modernen Medizin*, Münster - Hamburg - London: LIT.

Lilley, S. (2013) *Transhumanism and Society: The Social Debate over Human Enhancement*, Dordrecht - Heidelberg - New York - London: Springer.

Luber, B., Lisanby, S. H. (2014) Enhancement of human cognitive performance using transcranial magnetic stimulation (TMS), *NeuroImage* 85 (3), 961–970.

Lüthy, Ch. H. (2013) Historical and philosophical reflections on natural, enhanced and artificial man and women, in Koops, B. J., Lüthy, Ch. H., Nelis, A. (Eds) *Engineering the Human: Human Enhancement Between Fiction and Fascination*, Berlin - Heidelberg: Springer, 11–28.

Mauron, A. (2015) Choosing among possible persons: The ethics of prenatal selection in the postgenomic age, *Comptes Rendus Biologies* 338 (8–9), 566–570.

McGee, M. A. (2007) *A History of Man's Quest for Immortality*, Alabama: Fifth Estate.

McKenny, G. (2000) Human enhancement uses of biotechnology, ethics, therapy vs. enhancement, in Murray, T. H., Mehlman, M. J. (Eds) *Encyclopedia of Ethical, Legal, and Policy Issues in Biotechnology*, New York: John Wiley & Sons, Vol. I, 507–515.

McWhorter, L. (2009) Governmentality, biopower, and the debate over genetic enhancement, *Journal of Medicine and Philosophy* 34 (4), 409–437.

Mehlman, J. M. (2003) *Wondergenes: Genetic Enhancement and the Future of Society*, Bloomington: Indiana University Press.

Miller, P., Wilsdon, J. (2006) The man who wants to live forever, in Miller, P., Wilsdon, J. (Eds) *Better Humans? The Politics of Human Enhancement and Life Extension*, London: Demos, 51–58.

Miller, R. (2002) Extending life: Scientific prospects and political obstacles, *Milbank Quarterly* 80 (1), 155–174.

Nass, R. (2013) Growth hormone axis and aging, *Endocrinology and Metabolism Clinics in North America* 42 (2), 187–199.

Neugarten, B. L., Havighurst, R. J. (1977) *Extending the Human Life Span: Social Policy and Social Ethics*, Chicago: University of Chicago.

Olshansky, S. J. (Ed) (2016) *Aging: The Longevity Dividend*, New York: Cold Spring Harbor Laboratory Press.

Olshansky. S.J., Carnes, B. (2001) *The Quest for Immortality: Science at the Frontiers of Aging*, New York: Norton.

Overall, C. (2003) *Aging, Death, and Human Longevity: A Philosophical Inquiry*, Berkeley: University of California Press.

Overall, C. (2009) Life enhancement technologies and the significance of social category membership, in Savulescu, J., Bostrom, N. (Eds) *Human Enhancement*, Oxford - New York: Oxford University Press, 323–336.

Parens, E. (Ed) (1998a) *Enhancing Human Traits: Social and Ethical Implications*, Washington/DC: Georgetown University Press.

Parens, E. (1998b) Is better always good? Project on the prospect of technologies aimed at the enhancement of human capacities and traits, *Hastings Center Report* 28 (1), 1–17.

Parens, E. (2004) Enhancement uses of medical technology, in Post, S. G. (Ed) *Encyclopedia of Bioethics*, 3rd edition, New York – Detroit: Thomson, Macmillan Reference, Vol. II, 753–757.

Parens, E. (2009) Toward a more fruitful debate about enhancement, in Savulescu, J., Bostrom, N. (Eds) *Human Enhancement*, Oxford – New York: Oxford University Press, 177–194.

Passmore, J. A. (2000) *The Perfectibility of Man*, 3rd edition, Indianapolis: Liberty Fund.

Plotz, D. (2003) The ethics of enhancement: We can make ourselves stronger, fast, smarter. Should we? *Slate Magazine* (2003, March 12). Available at: www.slate.com/id/2079310 (Accessed 28/04/2017).

Rebrin, I., Foster, M. J., Sohal, R. S. (2011) Association between life-span extension by caloric restriction and thiol redox state in two different strains of mice, *Free Radical Biology and Medicine* 51 (1), 225–233.

Resnik, D. B. (2000) The moral significance of the therapy-enhancement distinction in human genetics, *Cambridge Quarterly of Healthcare Ethics* 9 (3), 365–377.

Rodriguez-Brenes, I. A., Peskin, C. S. (2010) Quantitative theory of telomere length regulation and cellular senescence, *Proceedings of the National Academy of Sciences of the United States of America* 107 (12), 5387-5392.

Roduit, J. A. R. (2016) *The Case for Perfection: Ethics in the Age of Human Enhancement*, New York: Peter Lang.

Sargent, M. G. (2005) *Biomedicine and the Human Condition. Challenges, Risks, and Rewards*, Cambridge – New York: Cambridge University Press.

Schwartz, P. H. (2005) Defending the distinction between treatment and enhancement, *American Journal of Bioethics* 5 (3), 17–19.

Savulescu, J. (2006) Justice, fairness, and enhancement, *Annales of the New York Academy of Sciences* 1093, 321–338.

Savulescu, J. (2001) Procreative beneficence: Why we should select the best children, *Bioethics* 15 (5–6), 413–426.

Selzer, M. (Ed) (1995) *The Impact of Increased Life Expectancy: Beyond the Grey Horizon*, New York: Springer.

Shapiro, H. M., Spece, R.G., Dresser, R., Clayton, E. W. (2003) *Bioethics and Law*, 2nd edition, St. Paul: Thomson, 1427–1486.

Smith, G. P. (2000) Genetic enhancement technologies and the new society, *Medical Law International* 4 (2), 85–95.

Sohal, R. and Weindruch, R. (1996) Oxidative stress, caloric restriction, and aging, *Science* 273 (5271), 59–63.

Stock, G. (2002) *Redesigning Humans: Our Inevitable Genetic Future*, New York: Houghton Mifflin.

Tauer, C. A. (2000) Human enhancement uses of biotechnology, ethics, human growth hormone, in Murray, T. M., Mehlman, M. J. (Eds) *Encyclopedia of Ethical, Legal, and Policy Issues in Biotechnology*, New York: John Wiley & Sons, Vol. I, 491–502.

Voss, L. D. (2001) Short normal stature and psychosocial disadvantage: A critical review of the evidence, *Journal of Pediatric Endocrinology and Metabolism* 14 (6), 701–711.

Wegman, M. P. et al. (2015) Practicality of intermittent fasting in humans and its effect on oxidative stress and genes related to aging and metabolism, *Rejuvenation Research* 18 (2), 162–172.

WHO (1946) *Constitution of the World Health Organization*. Available at http://www.who.int/en/ (Accessed 28/05/2017).

Wolpe, P. R. (2003) Treatment, enhancement, and the ethics of neurotherapeutics, *Brain and Cognition* 50 (3), 387–395.

Zaleski, C. G. (2004) In defense of immortality, in Post, S. G., Binstock, R. H. (Eds) *The Fountain of Youth. Cultural, Scientific, and Ethical Perspectives on Biomedical Goal*, Oxford – New York: Oxford University Press, 109–132.

Zou, Y., Tong, H. J., Li, M., Tan, K. S., Cao, T. (2017) Telomere length is regulated by FGF-2 in human embryonic stem cells and affects the life span of its differentiated progenies, *Biogerontology* 18 (1), 69–84.

Chapter 3

Transhumanism and immortality

Juraj Odorčák

Abstract: This chapter is a critical appraisal of the relationship between transhumanism and immortality. Immortality is accepted in transhumanism because it protects from the main badness of death, which is the absence of any possible enhancement. This chapter defines two kinds of immortality. These are then tested against two well-known philosophical arguments against immortality. Finally, it is argued that transhumanism is partially capable of refuting these objections to immortality.

Introduction

Who wouldn't want to be immortal? Agnes doesn't. But Laura, her sister, does. Laura can't understand why anyone wouldn't want to be immortal. Agnes can't understand why anyone would. Agnes and Laura live in perpetual conflict. Agnes gives up and dies. Laura wins. She takes Agnes's place, and dies too. In his novel *Immortality* Milan Kundera contemplates metaphorical immortality: People are alive so long as someone else remembers them (Kundera, 2006). Some people think not only about the memories of others but also about non-metaphorical immortality. This chapter is an analytical appraisal of the positive relation between transhumanism and immortality. In contrast to transhumanism, philosophy treats immortality with suspicion. Hence this chapter is an attempt to highlight both transhumanist and critical views of immortality. Laura and Agnes have both a role to play.

The first part of the chapter is devoted to defining transhumanism and its relation to immortality. It is a relation based on a negative appraisal of death. This critical view of death allows us to understand two different types of immortality. These types of immortality are then tested by philosophical arguments against immortality. In the last section of the chapter it is argued that transhumanism partly succeeds in refuting these objections. However, that does not mean that immortality is good. It could just mean that immortality (in the strong meaning) makes no sense.

Transhumanism

Transhumanism is an intellectual movement that argues in favour of (radical) human enhancement. Modern human enhancement is concerned with the deficiencies and limitations biologically inherent in humans (Tomašovičová, 2014, 462). A fundamental human limitation is temporality. If death means the end of human life, then it also means the end of an enhanced human life. That is why death is the greatest evil for transhumanism (More and More, 2013, 213). For N. Bostrom death is a tyrant that must be overcome (Bostrom, 2005, 273). A. Sandberg suggests that death is the greatest obstacle to happiness (Sandberg, 2013, 56). For A. de Grey death is simply repulsive (De Grey, 2013, 217). It is in this sense that immortality is a core ideal in transhumanism (Broderick, 2013, 434). M. More and N. Vita-More suggest that immortality is one of transhumanism's central values (More and Vita-More, 2013, 213). While N. Bostrom points out that the search for immortality was the main precursor to transhumanism (Bostrom, 2006, 64). According to M. Geddes the pursuit of immortality is a moral obligation (Geddes, 2004, 239). Some transhumanists even predict that immortality will be achieved in the next century (Best, 2004, 237). Other transhumanists suggest that immortality could have been achieved long ago had we given up on religion and focused on scientific knowledge (Minsky, 2013, 170). The assumption of immortality invokes a discussion on the technological capacity for immortality. The main candidates are human cyborgization (Kurzweil, 2013), genetic engineering (Magalhaes, 2004), advanced regenerative medicine (De Grey, 2008), therapeutic cloning (West, 2004), virtualization (mind uploading) (Koene, 2013), cryonics (Ettinger, 1966), nanomedicine (Freitas, 2004) or a combination of these different technologies (Rose, 2013, 201). Proponents point to some promising findings in gerontology research (De Grey, 2008, 25) and the expected results of technological progress (Rose, 2013, 204). Opponents suggest that there are natural biological limits of the human lifespan (Dong, Milholland and Vijg, 2016). However, the aim of this chapter is not to assess the debates on the technological feasibility of immortality. From the philosophical viewpoint, the sole belief in immortality is interesting. But before we can explore immortality, a more precise definition of the concept of death is required.

Death

In transhumanism death is understood as non-existence (More, 2013, 15). If one assumes that non-existence can be imagined, then there are various ways of doing so. Generally, it is assumed that death is in a certain sense the antithesis of life, the cessation and limit of life. The definition of death adopted in this chapter is: Death is the state of non-existence that occurs following the irreversible loss of an individual's life functions.

Admittedly this definition of death is not uncontroversial. The first problem is semantic. One can question whether non-existence can *be* a state. The familiar dispute over the referential and quantitative issues of negative existence would lead us into an extensive and complex discussion. We shall therefore leave them aside. Here we shall consider the state of non-existence in the intuitive and heuristic way of ordinary language.

The second problem is one of classification. If we accept that it is meaningful to refer to a state of non-existence, then we need to classify what that non-existence is. It is probable that we are not thinking of non-existence per se but of a particular type. For example, in the year 2017, the author of this chapter has no children. Hence his children are non-existent. That, however, does not mean that the author considers these non-existing children to be dead. The definition given above classifies death as a state that occurs *following* loss of life rather than *prior to* life. This temporalized perception of non-existence may not be acceptable to everyone.[1] This chapter is devoted to the problem of continuing life and to general perceptions of death, and so we shall leave aside the questions about the value of non-existence.

The next problem with the definition is that while it may be based on a widespread view of death, it is not the only view. The proposed definition hinges on the termination thesis of death. The termination thesis holds that death means the end of an individual's existence (Feldman, 2000, 100). In some religious and philosophical conceptions, however, the transformative thesis is advocated. The minimalist version of the transformative thesis holds that death is not the end but a transition to something *different*. The positive version of this thesis is concerned with identifying what that something *different* might be. But the transformative thesis is hard to accept from a transhumanist viewpoint. If (eternal) personal life exists af-

[1] For a discussion of the symmetry argument see, for example, Kaufman (2016).

ter death, then attempts at achieving immortality through technology are not only pointless but perhaps also damaging. Moreover, transhumanism tends towards naturalistic and scientific thinking. This kind of thinking (it seems) is generally based on the termination thesis of death rather than the transformative one.

The familiar problem with the criteria of death is another potentially problematic aspect of this definition. The question is which criteria point to the true loss of life functions. Having strict criteria is not unimportant. But the definition given above favours none of these criteria. It is not the precise moment at which death occurs that is important for immortality but whether it occurs at all. In this sense the definition is neutral on the criteria. What is important is whether the criteria point to a state that is irreversible. Many of the well-known criteria of death would appear to meet this condition.[2]

The last problem is a rhetorical one. In some cases, we talk of living people despite the fact they fulfil the definition of death. Aristotle is dead – but not entirely. Aristotle may no longer exist but his ideas do. In this sense Aristotle lives on through his work, in the same way as our dead predecessors live on in our memories of them. Expressions of this nature can have various social, emotional, psychological and other functions. We need to recognize though that their meaning is oppositional to the actual death of the person. Our dead predecessors are only metaphorically alive because they are truly dead. Transhumanism is about extending this true life not the metaphoric one.

These objections highlight a number of the problems with defining death. For us, however, death is interesting because of the way it is perceived in transhumanism. Transhumanists consider death to be an evil because of the absence of existence, the temporal persistence of death and the reality of death. A definition whereby death is the irreversible state of non-existence following the loss of a person's vital functions therefore probably suffices for the transhumanist view. Having clarified this conception of death we can move on to the problem of immortality.

[2] For an overview see, for instance, DeGrazia (2016, 80).

Immortality

In order to understand immortality one must first understand mortality. When we assume that we are mortal, we generally think that at some point in the future we will die. Mortality is therefore a dispositional property for death. We have already defined what death is so we can now arrive at a more precise definition of mortality. Mortality is an (living) individual's dispositional property for non-existence, which occurs during the irreversible loss of life functions. However, death can potentially occur in a variety of situations. At some point we will certainly die, but under certain circumstances it could happen at any time. This means that from the view of mortality we consider death to be both necessary and (variously) possible. This enables us to reveal two further refinements to the definition of mortality that capture our basic intuitions on mortality.

The first intuition assumes that death can occur at any moment. It would seem that each moment of our existence is endangered by the possibility of death. The conditioned nature of mortality means that death is possible at some future moment. Definition: Conditional mortality is an individual's dispositional property for the irreversible loss of existence at some future point. The second intuition assumes death must occur sometime. While we can we generally suppose that our death will necessarily occur at a specific moment in the future, in this supposition death is not a possibility but a necessity. Regardless of when we die, it is clear we will die sometime. Definition: Non-conditional mortality is an individual's dispositional property for the irreversible loss of existence at a specific moment. It would seem that humans are both conditionally and non-conditionally mortal. These conceptions of mortality are not entirely unproblematic, however.

The first problem concerns the difficulties of defining death. These were dealt with in the section on defining death and so we will not readdress them here. The second problem is categorical. The definitions of conditional and non-conditional mortality rely on the assumption that there are some dispositional properties. The idea that dispositional properties exist is a controversial one. The problem is that these properties indicate future realization (Goodman, 1983, 42). Recognizing the existence of such predicates could lead to other ontological links. This, though, does not necessarily mean that they cannot be used from the ordinary viewpoint.

Another potential problem concerns epistemology. How can we know that we are mortal? If death is non-existence, then we can hardly experience, know or feel death. It seems we can never know we are dead. This epistemological objection is based on the personal consequences of the termination thesis (Schumacher, 2011, 120). If we don't exist, then we can't know that we don't exist. But that doesn't mean that if we do exist, then we don't have good reason to suppose that at some time we won't exist. This knowledge is not innate, a priori or essential. We learn about death from experience. Experience tells us that many people are dead. None of them escaped death. If all these people are dead, then they must all have been mortal. Therefore, it is not entirely true that we cannot know death. We know it from thinking about our experiences, which in all probability point to the reality of our own mortality. We have entirely "good" reasons to suppose that there is such a thing as mortality.

Having clarified the conceptual framework and the problem of mortality we can move on to immortality. Immortality is evidently a property that means that a given person will not (somehow) die. It is therefore a dispositional property indicating that person will be able to prevent his or her death. Immortality is therefore the converse of mortality. We have already defined mortality, so we can now go on to define immortality. Immortality is an individual's dispositional property that protects against the non-existence that would occur following the irreversible loss of life functions.

Immortality is based on the negation of mortality. Mortality can be conditional, and non-conditional. The same is true of immortality which can be divided into conditional and non-conditional immortality.[3] Non-conditional immortality is an individual's dispositional property to necessary existence at all future moments. Irreversible loss of life functions is ruled out at all future moments. The individual will therefore be immortal at all future moments. Conditional immortality is individual's dispositional property to a possible existence at any future moment. Irreversible loss of life functions is ruled out at whichever future moment. The individual will be immortal at any future moment.

These forms of immortality may be similar, but they differ in one fundamental way. Where non-conditional immortality is concerned the individual will necessarily be alive at all future moments, but the conditionally immortal individual may be alive only at any future moment. Non-conditional immortality is thus irreversible and non-voluntary, while conditional immortality is reversible and voluntary. This distinction may seem marginal. But it may be crucial to the transhumanist desirability of immortality.

[3] A similar general approach to dividing immortality is defended by M. Burley. Burley separates immortality into necessary and contingent immortality (Burley, 2009, 541–543).

Immortality and the finiteness argument

There are approaches in philosophy in which it is argued that key aspects of our life hang on mortality. The loss of mortality, that is immortality, could therefore also mean the loss of life as valued by humans. Since the loss of life as valued by humans would not be beneficial, mortality is not bad, but in fact necessary and good. Arguments of this kind usually rely on human life having a definite timespan, on the finiteness of life. T. May for instance thinks that an infinitely long life would have no meaningful content for humans (May, 2009, 61). According to May meaningful activity is about favouring one activity over another. But favouring one activity over another only makes sense if the choices available are restricted in time or are finite. The fact that they are finite renders them meaningful. Infinity disqualifies meaningfulness. Immortality robs a person of a life with significant meaning (May, 2009, 62).

M. Nussbaum (Nussbaum, 1994) posits a similar argument. Nussbaum is not concerned with the loss of the meaning of life but with the loss of the value of life. It is an argument that is not simply an implicitly individualist one. According to Nussbaum mortality is essential to the human value system (Nussbaum, 1994, 226). By contrast immortality means the disappearance of any kind of meaningful value system; it means the death of values (Nussbaum, 1994, 226). An immortal life would lack various core values that shape the positive relationship people have with their own lives and with the lives of others. Nussbaum elaborates on this argument by listing specific values. These include courage, love, friendship, justice, restraint, self-sacrifice, compassion and other moral virtues (Nussbaum, 1994, 226). The specific examples are not perhaps that important. Generally the problem is: How can we respect life if we are immortal? If life truly could not come to an end, then all other values emanating from it would clearly be pointless, if not destroyed. The risk of death, mortality, therefore has a positive value.

These two arguments hinge on finiteness. In its general form the finiteness argument supposes that if immortality precludes any kind of finiteness, then it destroys the meaning of our life (May) or our entire value system (Nussbaum). Destroying the meaning of our life, or our value system, is unacceptable to us, so immortality would therefore not be acceptable. The transhumanist assumption about positive immortality need not be substantiated. On the contrary if this argument were truly valid then one could accuse transhumanism of having unarticulated negative consequences.

Let us look at the criticisms of this argument. The first transhumanist criticism might focus on the second assumption in the finiteness argument. Should we consider the loss of meaning and values to be unacceptable? The characteristic argument in transhumanism is that in the future new values will be created. Transhumanists are keen to emphasize that new technologies will mean that new suitable values and lifestyles will be required. They do not consider the destruction of the usual values or the traditional meaning of life to be necessarily bad.[4] One could consider destruction to be a beneficial acceleration of transhumanist efforts at human (and posthuman) enhancement. If the change in values does not concern us, then immortality may not either. The finiteness argument therefore needn't be seen as a threat to transhumanism and its belief in immortality.

However, this criticism of the finiteness argument does not adequately capture the problem. The problem is not the impossibility of replacing values but the inappropriacy of replacing human values. The validity of the argument does not preclude the possibility of a new value system being created. Quite the opposite, the persuasiveness of the finiteness argument lies in the problem of replacing, or destroying, the human system of values or meaning. Neither May nor Nussbaum rule out the idea that immortality may have value or meaning. Transhumanists can argue in favour of these other values. But if immortality means the substitution and end of human values, then one may question whether this kind of immortality is of value to humans. The finiteness argument does not therefore suggest that destroying the meaning of human life or of the human value system is unacceptable per se, but rather that is unacceptable to *us*.

It may therefore be appropriate to retain the meaning and values in some way. The loss of values and meaning depends on the first assumption of the finiteness argument. The second criticism of the finiteness argument should therefore focus on this first assumption. The first assumption states that if immortality precludes any kind of finiteness then it destroys the meaning of our life (May) or our value system (Nussbaum). The problem with this implication may be the antecedent. If the antecedent is not valid, then the consequence – the destruction of values and meaning – need not apply either. Immortality destroys the meaning of our life, or our value system, because it precludes any kind of finiteness. The validity of this statement is therefore crucially dependent on the form of immortality assumed.

---

[4] This debate generally relates to the transhumanist perception of human nature as well. The transhumanist rejection of human nature is criticised both from a communal (Sitarčíková, 2012) and a secular perspective (Sýkora, 2014).

In the previous section we defined non-conditional and conditional immortality. Non-conditional immortality implies an individual's existence at all future moments. An immortal person thus conceived of must live forever. There are no circumstances, and there is no situation, under which loss of life functions could occur. This kind of immortality is total, absolute, irreversible and necessarily infinite. Since this kind of immortality is necessarily infinite, it has to preclude the possibility of any kind of finiteness. The assumption that immortality is non-conditional therefore unquestionably underpins the antecedent of the first premise of the infinity argument. If the immortality assumed is this form of immortality, then the idea about the destruction of values may be valid.

But transhumanism is not necessarily bound to the validity of this form of immortality. A conditionally immortal person may be alive at any future moment. But that means he or she need not be alive at some future moments. This kind of immortal person may, but need not, live forever. Conditional immortality is therefore not necessarily infinite. If it is not necessarily infinite, then this kind of immortality does not preclude the possibility of the end or finiteness. Conditional immortality allows this possibility, and so there is no obligation to assume the consequences of the implication of the first assumption. The destruction of the values and meaning of life in the finiteness argument hinges upon the complete elimination of the possibility of death. Our value system or the search for meaning is based on the risk of death. Not only those who necessarily die live with this risk, but also those who may die, that is, conditionally immortal people. It is perhaps true that non-conditional immortality leads to the destruction of the meaning of life and its values. But conditional immortality does not necessarily lead to this conclusion, and so this finiteness argument is not entirely accurate.

Transhumanism may therefore partially cast doubt on the validity of the finiteness argument. Absolute, total, non-voluntary immortality is not necessarily acceptable to people, as this finiteness argument indicates. The assumption of this non-conditional immortality is nonetheless problematic, if not directly inconsistent.[5] On the other hand, the finite argument does not necessarily disqualify conditional immortality. It is therefore much better for transhumanism to assume this second kind of immortality. The finiteness argument is therefore not necessarily valid. It appears that immortality could be acceptable. Perhaps, though, the problem is not whether immortality is acceptable but whether it is desirable.

[5] For example: What would the non-conditional immortal *do* in the case of the heath death of universe?

The Makropulos Case

The Makropulos Case is a play by the writer Karel Čapek (Čapek, 2015). It is about the immortality of the main protagonist, Elina Makropulos. The opera by Leoš Janáček based on this play was the inspiration for the well-known argument about the undesirability of immortality. The argument was developed by B. Williams (Williams, 1973). Like the previous argument this one highlights the fact that immortality is not necessarily beneficial since human mortality provides meaningfulness. The difference is that Williams's argument does not concern values per se, but the value of personal immortality.

The plot of the Makropulos Case opens with Makropulos, a Rudolphine alchemist, discovering an elixir for immortality. Makropulos offers the elixir to his daughter Elina. Elina takes it and becomes immortal. For centuries she travels around Europe, searching for love, success and fulfilment. In the end, however, she discovers that she believes in none of these and envies mortal beings for their naïve, but meaning giving beliefs. She therefore decides to return to where it all began. She goes back to Prague and terminates her immortality.

Williams thinks Elina's decision is understandable. The problem with immortality is the threat of existential emptiness. Williams's argument is based on the idea that if we were truly immortal, then we would think immortality was unpleasant and absurd. Williams reaches this position via two stages. First he addresses the problem that death is bad. He believes death is bad because it sometimes prevents us from fulfilling our resolutions, desires and projects. The loss of the ability to implement these projects is bad, and so it is reasonable to consider death to be bad as well (Williams, 1973, 82). Cautiousness of death and delaying death are justified. Williams does not therefore doubt that death is bad, he considers it to be a fact.

In stage two Williams points out that the fear of death doesn't imply that immortality is desirable or that mortality is negative. Elina may have considered death to be bad; however, that did not prevent her from envying the mortality of others or regretting her own immortality. The understandable attempt to delay death need not mean postponing it indefinitely. On the contrary, immortality, at least for Elina, appears to be a worse option than mortality and death. But why did Elina ultimately choose to end her immortality? The postponement of death is, Williams posits, justifiable if death will prevent that person from realizing projects and desires they consider beneficial. Elina had undertaken all her projects and had come to understand their meaningfulness or naivety. This is why she ultimately surrendered to resignation and cynism, and made her final decision. Elina had achieved all that she wanted and her life had subsequently become empty, boring and unbearable.

The same argument can be made in a less metaphorical format. Williams's criticism of immortality is based on two assumptions: A desirable life must be one that maintains that person's life; a desirable life means realizing projects the person considers important. Immortality is undesirable because it does not allow that person to maintain his life, or if it does, then it leads to the exhaustion of all meaningful projects. Either we don't have personal immortality or we have an unbearably exhausting personal immortality. In either case this kind of immortality is not desirable from the individual viewpoint. Williams's argument exceeds the finiteness argument. The assumption that immortality destroys the usual values is perhaps not so important. What is important is that immortality could destroy the person. If this were true, nobody with any common sense should choose immortality. The transhumanist attempt at immortality would therefore be irrational.

Williams's argument is not unproblematic. Most of his criticism is aimed at the second assumption, that of the project problem. One may question which projects are important to people. Clearly not all projects are of equal value. Williams therefore distinguishes between conditional and categorical desires (Williams, 1973, 86). Categorical desires are projects that give meaning to our lives. Conditional desires simply sustain our lives momentarily. Williams supposes that immortality will ultimately rob us of these categorical desires. His critics have concentrated on the appropriacy of this distinction (Fischer, 1994, 260), on the nature of categorical desires (Bradley and McDaniel, 2013, 120) and on the possibility of renewing categorical desires (Bruckner, 2012, 629). We can leave this problem aside. Immortality will necessarily lead to the exhaustion of all meaningful projects only if immortality is infinite, non-conditional. This type of immortality was rejected in the previous section and so we shall look at the first assumption in Williams's argument.

The first assumption concerns the problem of identity. The assumption that a desirable life must retain that person's life is trivial. Immortality could then be good (or bad) for us if it is our own immortality.[6] Williams

[6] This assumption does not mean that the person is necessarily interested only in their own immortality. Being interested in one's own good does not preclude an interest in the good of others or even an interest in the good per se. On this reading Williams's argument is not tied to an egocentric or selfish moral model.

assumes that if immorality lasts a sufficiently long time then personal identity is under threat. However, that depends on the type of identity. In this case Williams is not thinking of identity in the robust metaphysical sense. Metaphysical conceptions of identity are concerned with the conditions under which objects generally persist. These conditions can be formulated in various ways. With a certain degree of liberalness one could imagine a conception that metaphysically underpins the identity of some eternal or immortal object. Williams was not thinking about the biological identity of a person either. For him, Elina was, in terms of identity, one and the same person biologically (Williams, 1973, 92). The problem lies in a different kind of identity, a practical (psychological) identity. According to this conception of identity, a person is the same practically speaking if certain psychological characteristics are maintained over time.

In practical terms we often use and examine this identity. For instance, sometimes we accept the idea that a person becomes a new person following a transformative experience. It seems that for Williams immortality is one of the most radical transformative experiences. This is because with infinity the possibility of change increases endlessly and with it comes the demise of the original person. The paradox of immortality lies in choosing our own possible demise. That is not a good prospect. Hence choosing immortality ceases to be desirable for that person.

Williams's assumption could be incorrect for two reasons. It is based on practical identity but Williams does not break it down any further. It should be noted that we usually consider this identity when we are thinking about decisions that affect our personal future. We think about whether some decision will lead to our psychological characteristics being maintained in the long run. We generally wish to be the same in the future.[7] We could call this kind of practical identity prospective practical identity. We consider prospective practical identity when judging future changes to the person. But this is not the only way of thinking about practical identity. Sometimes we look backwards instead of forwards. We retrospectively judge whether our decisions ultimately led to our current psychological characteristics. When we consider retrospective practical identity, we assess changes to the person in the past.

These two kinds of practical identity can lead to different outcomes in Williams's identity problem. In the prospective one it could seem that over a sufficient length of time the person could change psychologically, or po-

[7] This is not always the case. One could argue that some decisions are about changing and not retaining that person. However, we will leave this criticism aside.

tentially cease to exist. However, this needn't apply to the retrospective one. In fact the future immortal person may be grateful for having opted for immortality in the past. Generally, in the retrospective approach many of the changes to our personality, desires, wishes, longings may seem to be the right ones even when they didn't on the prospective view. It may even seem that we have become the person we are today because of these changes. That does not mean that immortality isn't necessarily unpleasant. It simply means that identity could be safeguarded on the retrospective reading. However, it should be recognized that on the prospective reading this is not necessarily the case.

This brings us to the second problem with the assumption of identity. Why is identity not safeguarded on the prospective reading? The potential for unacceptable personal changes increases over the course of an infinitely long life. But this again depends on the kind of immortality we are talking about. Non-conditional immortality can only mean living for all infinity. Having to live forever endlessly increases the potential for personal change. This kind of immortality is also hard to accept for various other reasons. Williams uses Elina as his example, but her immortality is not a given. Her immortality can end; it is conditional. Conditional immortality does not lead to an ever higher likelihood of personal change. If we suppose that immortality is conditional, then the fears inherent in the prospective problem of identity need not be substantiated.

Williams's argument operates on two levels. The first assumption is based on the identity problem and the second is based on the project problem. The negativity of immortality lies in the fact that it may not necessarily end up being our personal immortality or that it will be an exhausting personal immortality. If these premises are valid, then the transhumanist arguments favouring immortality are not substantiated or beneficial. However, transhumanism has the potential to avoid these consequences. The force of the argument is weakened by the fact that it could point to a different type of immortality and a different type of identity. Conditional immortality does not fully prevent all important projects from being exhausted. It is possible to imagine an immortality in which there is sufficient time for people to pursue, implement and renew their projects. Similarly, Williams's assumption of identity is weakened by a different type of practical identity. A retrospective practical identity does not preclude the possibility that the identity of a conditionally immortal person is safeguarded. Transhumanism is therefore capable of refuting both the finiteness argument and Williams's argument against immortality.

However, none of this means that immortality is good.

Conclusion

It has been shown that transhumanism has the capacity to demonstrate that fears of immortality are not necessarily valid. However, the fact that they are not necessarily valid does not mean that they are unsubstantiated. The finiteness argument and Williams's argument point to various complications with immortality. The finiteness argument indicates that immortality can in certain cases lead to negative social consequences. Williams's argument shows that the problem with personal immortality is the inherent risk of an exhausting and absurd personal emptiness.

Doubt can be cast on both arguments by highlighting the fact that there are imaginable conceptions of a different kind of immortality and a different kind of identity which need not lead to negative consequences. Only non-conditional immortality will necessarily destroy the value system. It is also the only kind of immortality that will necessarily lead to the emptiness and demise of the person. Conditional immortality does not necessarily rule out the persistence of values or the person. But that does not mean that conditional immortality necessarily excludes the possibility of destruction of values or persons. And this is precisely the problem with the debate on immortality.

One can imagine that an almost infinite and therefore also a conditionally immortal life could lead to alienation from human values and meaning. Similarly, one can imagine that this type of conditionally immortal life thus could ultimately lead to exhaustion and loss of a person's authenticity. As a person's conditionally immortal life progressed, this could become likely. The problem is not infinity, the problem is the amount of time. The crucial point with the whole problem of so-called immortality in transhumanism is that it centres around the controversy over the acceptable length of conditional immortality. Ultimately conditional immortality is perhaps not immortality but rather a long-lasting form of mortality. Thus the real debate is not about immortality but about what is a good and tolerable length of human life, human longevity. This is not a trivial question, and the possible normative aspects are certainly complex. It is possible that Elina may be robbed of her values in precisely three hundred years; it is also possible that Methuselah may not have lost his values even after 968 years. However, in the end none of this changes the implication that immortality is not a de facto problem, because immortality in the absolute (non-conditional) sense seems to be potentially absurd. Transhumanism would therefore do best and leave the talk about immorality where it belongs. But where is true immortality?

Acknowledgement

This work was supported by Slovak Research and Development Agency contract No. APVV-0379-12.

Literature

Best, B. (2004) Some problems with immortalism, in Immortality institute (ed.) *The scientific conquest of death*, Buenos Aires: LibrosEnRed, 233–238.

Bostrom, N. (2005) The fable of the dragon tyrant, *Journal of medical ethics* 31(5), 273–276.

Bostrom, N. (2006) A short history of transhumanist thoughts, *Analysis and metaphysics* 5 (1–2), 63–95.

Bradley, B. and McDaniel, K. (2013) Death and desires, in Taylor, J. C. (Ed) *The metaphysics and ethics of death: New essays*, Oxford: Oxford University Press, 118–133.

Broderick, D. (2013) Trans and post, in More, M. and Vita-More, N. (Eds) *The transhumanist reader*, Malden: Wiley-Blackwell, 430–437.

Bruckner, D. W. (2012) Against the tedium of immortality, *Journal of philosophical studies* 20 (5), 623–644.

Burley, M. (2009) Immortality and meaning: Reflections on the Makropulos debate, *Philosophy* 84 (330), 529–547.

Čapek, K. (2015) *Věc Makropulos*, Praha: Artur.

DeGrazia, D. (2014) The nature of human death, in Luper, S. (Ed) *The Cambridge companion to life and death*, New York: Cambridge University Press, 80–97.

De Grey, A. (2013) The curate's egg of anti-anti-aging bioethics, in More, M. and Vita-More, N. (Eds) *The transhumanist reader*, Malden: Wiley-Blackwell, 215–219.

De Grey, A. and Rae, M. (2008) *Ending aging*, New York: St. Martin's press.

Dong, X., Milholland, B. and Vijg, J. (2016) Evidence for a limit to human lifespan, *Nature* 538, 257–259.

Ettinger, R. C. W. (1966) *The prospect of immortality*, New York: McFadden - Bartell.

Feldman, F. (2000) The termination thesis, *Midwest studies in philosophy* 24 (1), 98–115.

Fischer, J. M. (1994) Why immortality is not so bad, *International journal of philosophical studies* 2 (2), 257–270.

Freitas, R. A. (2004) Nanomedicine, in Immortality institute (Ed) *The scientific conquest of death*, Buenos Aires: LibrosEnRed, 77–92.

Geddes, M. (2004) An introduction to immortalist morality, in Immortality institute (Ed) *The scientific conquest of death*, Buenos Aires: LibrosEnRed, 239–256.

Goodman, N. (1983) *Fact, fiction and forecast*, Cambridge: Harvard University Press.

Kaufman, F. (2016) Lucretius and the fear of death, in Colby, M. (Ed) *Immortality and the philosophy of death*, New York: Rowman and Littlefield, 53–66.

Koene, R. A. (2013) Uploading to substrate-independent minds, in More, M. and Vita-More, N. (Eds) *The transhumanist reader*, Malden: Wiley-Blackwell, 146–156.

Kundera, M. (2016) *Nesmrtelnost*, Brno: Atlantis.

Kurzweil, R. (2004) Human body version 2.0, in Immortality institute (Ed), *The scientific conquest of death*, Buenos Aires: LibrosEnRed, 93–106.

Magalhaes, J. P. (2004) The dream of elixir vitae, in Immortality institute (Ed) *The scientific conquest of death*, Buenos Aires: LibrosEnRed, 47–62.

May, T. (2009) *Death*, Stocksfield: Acumen.

Minsky, M. (2013) Why Freud was the first good AI theorist, in More, M. and Vita-More, N. (Eds) *The transhumanist reader*, Malden: Wiley-Blackwell, 167–176.

More, M. (2013) The philosophy of transhumanism, in More, M. and Vita-More,V. (Eds) *The transhumanist reader*, Malden: Wiley-Blackwell, 3–17.

More, M. and Vita-More, N. (2013) Engines of life: Identity and beyond death, in More, M. and Vita-More, N. (Eds) *The transhumanist reader*, Malden: Wiley-Blackwell, 213–215.

Nussbaum, M. C. (1994) *The therapy of desire*, Princeton: Princeton University Press.

Rose, M. R. (2013) Immortalist fictions and strategies, in More, M. and Vita-More, N. (Eds) *The transhumanist reader*, Malden: Wiley-Blackwell, 196–204.

Sandberg, A. (2013) Morphological freedom – Why we not just want it, but need it, in More, M. and Vita-More, V. (Eds) *The transhumanist reader*, Malden: Wiley-Blackwell, 56–64.

Schumacher, B. (2011) *Death and mortality in contemporary philosophy*, New York: Cambridge University Press.

Sitarčíková, Z. (2012) *O šľachtení človeka: Nanotechnológie, transhumanizmus a ľudská prirodzenosť*, Trnava: Typi Universitatis Tyrnaviensis.

Sýkora, P. (2014) Kritika teologicko-teleologickej koncepcie ľudskej prirodzenosti ako dôvodu odmietnutia transhumanizmu, *Filozofia* 69 (6), 514–525.

Tomašovičová, J. (2014) Život v zóne biomoci: Etický a biopolitický diskurz o transhumanizme, *Filozofia* 69 (6), 461–471.

West, M. D. (2004) Therapeutic cloning, in Immortality institute (Ed) *The scientific conquest of death*, Buenos Aires: LibrosEnRed, 63–76.

Williams, B. (1973) The Makropulos case: Reflections on the tedium of immortality, in Williams, B. (Ed) *Problems of the self*, New York: Cambridge University Press, 82–100.

Chapter 4

Can we use the capabilities approach to evaluate human enhancement?

Ivars Neiders

Abstract: The main task of this chapter is to evaluate the proposal made by Johann Roduit that Nussbaum's capability approach (CA) can be used to assess morality of human enhancement. Roduit claims that the capabilities approach is a type-perfectionist theory that can be used both as guiding and restricting human enhancement. I argue that the claim about using CA for guiding relies on the assumption that the central capabilities can be maximized, but this assumption is problematic. Moreover, many capabilities on Nussbaum's list of the central capabilities are such that they cannot be affected by biomedical means. A closer examination of CA shows that it provides no incentives for human enhancement. Of course, CA can still be used as restricting; however, in that case one must be careful to take into account the distinction between capabilities and functionings, and this seems to be ignored in Roduit's account.

Introduction

If you were offered a chance to live a longer life (and not just few years longer, but considerably longer, let's say, three or four times longer than the current average lifespan) would you take the offer? And what about your cognitive abilities or physical strength? If by using some, let's assume, safe biomedical technologies it would be possible to improve them well beyond the levels that people currently enjoy, would you go for it? Well, it might turn out that you would, but would that be the right thing to do? What are the moral implications of using biomedical technologies for enhancing ourselves? In the bioethical literature this is often referred to as the problem of moral permissibility of human enhancement.[1] There are different camps of bioethicists arguing pro or contra ethical permissibility of enhancing humans. To formulate their different takes on the permissibility of human enhancement various moral frameworks are used by the authors. Some refer to safety, some to justice, autonomy, human nature, authenticity, etc.[2] Recently, some authors (e.g., Roduit, 2016)[3] have suggested that the best framework to assess morality of human enhancement is Martha

[1] In fact, there is still no consensus about how enhancement should be defined, but I will avoid this thorny issue here. For a useful recent discussion see Gyngell and Selgelid 2016. See also Savulescu, 2013, Menuz, Hurlimann, Godard, 2013.

[2] For a good overview and further references see Roduit, Helinger, Baumann, 2015.

[3] See also Hughes, 2011, and Coeclekbergh, 2011.

Nussbaum's capability approach (CA).[4] In short, CA is a theoretical framework about human well-being and justice. One of the main claims of the approach is that achievement of well-being is a matter of what people are able to do and to be. The capabilities, according to Nussbaum, are answers to this question (Nussbaum, 2011, 18). Nussbaum gives a list of ten central capabilities which include life, bodily health; bodily integrity; senses, imagination, and thought; emotions; practical reason; affiliation; other species; play; and control over one's environment.

The main task of this chapter is to evaluate Johan Roduit's version of such a proposal. In the next section, I describe Roduit's position and his reasons for proposing it. Then I turn to the discussion. First, I address the question, whether CA can deliver what Roduit claims it can. Second, I discuss the question whether CA as such provides any incentives for human enhancement.

Roduit on the capabilities approach and human enhancement

According to Roduit, the concept of perfection is unavoidable in the debate of the ethics of human enhancement. Roduit claims that despite the appearances the participants of the enhancement debate, both so-called bioconservatives and bioliberals implicitly rely on some conception of perfection. This might seem paradoxical especially in the case of bioconservatives who have been rather explicit that there is something morally wrong about striving for perfection allegedly defended by bioliberal authors. However, Roduit convincingly shows that this explicit hostility towards perfection does not rule out the reliance on a particular conception of perfection (Roduit, 2016, 60–63). This becomes obvious as soon as we observe the distinction between the concept of perfection and different conceptions of perfection. To illustrate the point, let us consider the case of Michael Sandel. In his book titled *The Case Against Perfection* (Sandel, 2007)[5], Sandel famously opposes the use of genetic technologies to perfect our nature. He considers enhancement objectionable because:

---

[4] Capabilities Approach originally was introduced by Amartya Sen and further developed by many other authors, e.g. Martha Nussbaum.

[5] The title of Roduit's book *The Case for Perfection* should, of course, be taken as an answer to that of Sandel's.

> It expresses and entrenches a certain stance toward the world – a stance of mastery and dominion that fails to appreciate the gifted character of human powers and achievements, and misses the part of freedom that consists in a persisting negotiation with the given. (Ibid. 83)

Roduit, however, correctly points out that Sandel's stance should not be seen as being against the idea of perfection. It is rather a stance against a certain form of perfection that Sandel considers to be flawed. Moreover, Sandel himself, albeit implicitly, uses his own assumptions about perfection to argue against those that he considers to be morally unacceptable. As Roduit (Roduit, 2016, 61) puts it:

> For Sandel, the 'perfect' human being should strive to develop the virtues of humility, solidarity, responsibility and gratitude, because this is a "proper stance of human beings towards the given world". (Sandel, 2007, 9)

These are the ideals that according to Sandel are threatened by genetic engineering and other enhancement technologies. So, it turns out that Sandel is not against perfection after all. He just has a different idea of it.

Similar considerations, according to Roduit, apply to bioliberals, e.g., John Harris, Allan Buchanan[6] (Roduit, 2016, 63–66). On the one hand, bioliberals have been very skeptical about the concept of perfection. Roduit mentions two reasons for such attitude. First, bioliberals don't think that the concept of perfection is relevant for the enhancement debate. In their account enhancement is not about perfection but about improvement of human functioning. From that point of view all the objections against enhancement conceived as striving for perfection are misguided. Second, bioliberals have objected against the concept of perfection on normative grounds. As people have different conceptions of perfection, it would be wrong in a liberal society to impose one view of perfection on all individuals. However, on the other hand, according to Roduit, despite the points just mentioned, bioliberals also implicitly endorse a certain conception of perfection. Roduit argues that

> If they are only concerned with moral constraints on enhancements, and leave it up to individuals to decide whether to engage in enhancement, this indeed presupposes some ideal of (individual) mastery over human nature (i.e. regarded distorted by bioconservatives). This is based on a strong understanding of an

[6] See Harris, 2007, Buchanan, 2011.

individual's *autonomy*, a concept that figures prominently within the bioliberals ideal of a human life. (Ibid. 65)

Roduit's argument here seems less persuasive than in the case of bioconservatives, as a commitment to the principle of autonomy by itself does not imply a commitment to any particular ideal of human life. Nevertheless, for argument's sake let's assume that he is right.

Roduit's main point so far is that as far as the enhancement debate is concerned the concept of perfection deserves serious attention. Now the question is, how to decide which particular conception of perfection should we choose? To answer this question Roduit comes up with three criteria that a satisfactory conception should satisfy (Ibid. 31). First, it must provide an objective ideal of what human being ought to be. Second, it should be flexible enough to allow room for pluralism and political deliberation. Finally, it should provide not only restriction but guidance as well. Roduit claims that the best available conception that satisfies all the above-mentioned criteria is the capabilities approach developed by Martha Nussbaum in a series of papers and monographs.

In what follows, I argue that Roduit is wrong and CA is less useful as an account of perfection in the enhancement debate than Roduit likes to think. But before presenting my objections, let's see why Roduit thinks that CA satisfies the criteria.

Why the capabilities approach?

Following Walker, Roduit distinguishes two conceptions of perfection: type-perfection and property-perfection. Type-perfection is the thesis that the ideal of perfection is best exemplified by those individuals who best realize the properties of the type that the individual belongs to. Property-perfection on the other hand is the thesis that the ideal of perfection is best exemplified by those individuals who best realize some property or set of properties (Roduit, 2016, 89). Proponents of type-perfection accept enhancement within limits of a type. Proponents of property-perfection accept enhancement of any function without making reference to any given type. The following example will clarify the concepts. Consider a proposal to enhance the cognitive capacities of a chimp. Proponents of type-perfectionism will say that the cognitive abilities of a chimp should be improved only as far as the chimp remains a chimp and does not turn into a different type of animal. For proponents of property-perfectionism this is not an issue. They would say that we should try to perfect the cognitive abilities of a chimp as far as we can even if that means turning the chimp into a sort of post-chimp.

Further, Roduit points out that ideas about perfection may come from two different sources: the subjective view and the objective view (Ibid. 91, Roduit, Heilinger, Baumann, 2015, 624–625). According to the subjective view one's type-perfection or property-perfection is subjective. It may be a list of subjective goods. From this point of view enhancement should be defined according to individuals. According the objective view the ideals of type-perfection or property-perfection are objective.

Roduit argues that property-perfectionism is flawed because it falls back on type-perfectionist view. His main contention is that property-perfectionism is an incomplete view, because properties are always associated with a type:

> For example, when we speak of the perfect speed, we do so in reference to a certain type, such as an athlete. The property of speed has to be embodied in a type, which could of course take different forms such as a human, a posthuman, another species or even the form of an object. In all of these examples it is embodied in a type. (Ibid. 90)[7]

Therefore, the preferred conception of perfection should be a version of type-perfectionism. Further, Roduit argues that type-perfectionism in turn implies a commitment to objectivity as the very nature of type is that it is shared (Ibid. 93–94, Roduit, Heilinger, Baumann, 2015, 626). This means that we are left with a notion of an objective type-perfectionism. Moreover, the reason we need a conception of perfection is that the conception should fulfill two functions: it should function both as a constraint of human enhancement and as a guiding principle (Roduit, 2016, 95, Roduit, Heilinger, Baumann, 2015, 626–627).

After considering various types of perfectionist conceptions (Roduit, 2016, 96–102), Roduit claims that the most promising objective type-perfectionist conception that can serve both as a constraint and as a guide of human enhancement is Nussbaum's capabilities approach. First, Roduit takes capabilities as an objective list of goods that define an ideal human (Ibid. 107). In this he follows Coeckelbergh's (Coeckelbergh, 2011, 82) claim

[7] See also Roduit, Heilinger, Baumann, 2015, 624.

that the "central capabilities can be interpreted as an expression of what it is to be human". Therefore, says Roduit:

> The ideal human (towards which we are striving with human enhancement) should have those capabilities. A set of enhanced central capabilities can thus be interpreted as an expression of an enhanced human. (Roduit, 2016, 107)

Roduit describes CA as an objective theory; however, he does not specify further how this notion should be understood. It is worth noticing that this is not Nussbaum's preferred way of presenting the approach. In her later expositions of the theory, 'objectivity' is not mentioned at all. Instead of that she talks about defending a set of universal values (see e.g., Nussbaum, 2000). In her earlier presentations of the theory (e.g., Nussbaum, 1988), however, CA is described as objective. Here she says that the approach should be on the one hand non-detached, but on the other hand, objective. By saying that the theory should be non-detached she means that:

> It should not be discovered by looking at human lives and actions from a totally alien point of view, outside of the conditions and experience of those lives - as if we were discovering some sort of value-neutral scientific fact about ourselves. (Nussbaum, 1988a, 174-75)

But the approach is still objective in the sense that: "We do not want simply to take each culture's or group's word for it, when they tell us what they think the relevant human functionings are - even when they are talking about themselves" (ibid.) In other words, objectivity is required for the approach to have the power to criticize views that are, for example, biased by some customs or traditions. Later in *Women and Human Development* Nussbaum describes CA as a middle ground position between two extremes. One the one hand, there is what she calls *subjective welfarism* that holds that all existing preferences are of equal status. On the other extreme, there is *Platonism* that holds that given the unreliability of desires and preferences as guides to what is really good, they should not be taken as having any relevance. What we do need instead is an argument for an objective set of values that is independent of people's desires and preferences (Nussbaum, 2000, 116–17). Although both views are motivated by genuine concerns, Nussbaum argues that they are problematic as the subjective welfarism forces us to accept any preferences, but Platonism makes human preferences irrelevant. She presents the capabilities as "the object of overall consensus among people who otherwise have very different comprehensive conceptions of the good" (Nussbaum, 2006, 70).[8] The list of the capabilities, according to Nussbaum, is the "outgrowth of a process of critical normative argument, centrally involving the notion of human dignity" (Nussbaum, 2011, 108).

Thus, we can agree with Roduit that Nussbaum's proposal satisfies two of the above-mentioned conditions. It is in a sense objective, but not in a Platonic way as it takes into account people's preferences. And it is at the same time flexible, because the capacities are defined in somewhat abstract and general way so that they can be implemented in number of different ways. How particular capabilities are interpreted and implemented should be the outcome of democratic deliberation of particular society in question (Nussbaum, 2000, 77, Nussbaum, 2011, 108). To illustrate this point Nussbaum uses and example of the different approaches to freedom of speech in Germany and the USA. So, the German ban on all anti-Semitic writing would be considered as too restrictive for the USA, but provided the different historical circumstances in both countries, the differences in the scope of freedom of speech makes sense.

So far so good. However, I have some issues with Roduit's third criterion. In what follows, I show that unfortunately for Roduit's account, CA fails to satisfy it.

Restriction and guidance

Roduit claims that one of the advantages of CA is that it - unlike other type-perfectionist views - can be used both for restricting and for guiding:

> On the one hand, it is constraining because a given enhancement that would cause one to fall under the threshold of a central capability would be seen as morally problematic. At the same time, it is guiding because a given enhancement should move a human towards a holistic ideal human, as outlined by the central capabilities. (Roduit, 2016, 110)

It seems to me that Roduit is wrong here and the main reason for that is his misunderstanding of Nussbaum's account. First of all, it looks like

[8] See also Nussbaum, 2011, 93.

Roduit misunderstands the purpose of CA. In more than one place Nussbaum has stressed that the main intention of CA is to specify some necessary conditions for a decently just society:

> The capabilities approach is a political doctrine about basic entitlements, not a comprehensive moral doctrine. It does not even claim to be a complete political doctrine, since it simply specifies some necessary conditions for a decently just society, in the form of a set of fundamental entitlements of all citizens. (Nussbaum, 2006, 155)

In short, in Nussbaum's version CA is used to construct a theory of basic social justice (Nussbaum, 2011, 19), and the central capabilities are supposed to be general goals that constitute part of a minimum account of social justice. It is only part of the theory as it specifies only some necessary conditions of just society. And it is part of a minimum account, because it specifies some threshold conditions of justice and life worth of human dignity. Roduit, however, talks about 'ideal human', which seems to be a considerably higher aim than Nussbaum's minimum. Roduit seems to be aware of this mismatch of the goals of both theories as he agrees with Coeckelbergh (Roduit, 2016, 109), who points out, that:

The capabilities can be understood not only as *minimal* requirements or 'thresholds' for dignity or justice, as Nussbaum usually sees them, but rather as formulations of ethical 'maximum': they can be interpreted as what good life or human *flourishment* requires. (Coeckelbergh, 2011, 84)

Roduit, following Coeckelbergh's suggestion, assumes that the central capabilities are an expression of what it is to be human. Thus, an enhanced human is a human with a set of enhanced central capacities (Roduit, 2016, 107). Unfortunately, there are at least two problems with this claim. First, Coeckelbergh's interpretation of the CA is not entirely correct. Second, it relies on a dubious assumption that the central capacities allow maximization. Let us look into both problems in order.

In her presentation of the CA Nusbaum in fact discusses the distinction between two different thresholds (Nussbaum, 1992, 221, Nussbaum, 1995, 81):

1) HUMAN LIFE THRESHOLD (HLT): A threshold of capability to function, beneath which a life will be so impoverished that it will not be human at all.
2) GOOD HUMAN LIFE THRESHOLD (GHLT): A threshold, beneath which those characteristic functions are available in such a reduced way that although we may judge the form of life a human one, we will not think of it a *good* human life.

Nussbaum admits that albeit it is not an easy task to determine where each threshold is located on the continuum of abilities, one still can describe some cases where existence is so impoverished that it cannot be properly called human life. As primary examples of such condition Nussbaum mentions existence that many people suffer at the end of their lives when the being that has survived has permanently lost the capacity of sensation, consciousness, or the capacity to recognize loved ones, to think and to reason, etc. (Ibid., 82). It is important to notice that when Nussbaum addresses the question about which threshold should societies to aim for their citizens it is GHLT and not HLT that she endorses. In other words, CA is intended as an account of the second threshold. Now it should be clear that the claim that the capabilities express what it means to be human doesn't do justice to Nussbaum's account. According to Nusbaum, bare human life is already captured by HLT. Further, Coeckelbergh's implication that the capabilities are not taken by Nussbaum as conditions for good human life is wrong as well, as Nussbaum explicitly says the opposite.

Now, one may try to defend Roduit and suggest the following: Let us grant that CA already intends to capture the threshold for good human life, but it is still possible to aim at some higher threshold for a better human life, and this threshold then should serve as our guide for human enhancement. This brings us to our second problem.

I already pointed out that Roduit assumes that within the framework of CA to enhance means to maximize the central capabilities (Roduit, 2016, 107).[9] This, however, is not that simple. Roduit further specifies that this does not mean that just maximizing the central capacities would be considered as enhancement for the simple reason that maximization of one capacity over another might be counterproductive, as enhancement of one capability might destroy or impede another capability. For this reason, Roduit suggests we should "maximize all capabilities together as a harmonious, holistic set" (Ibid. 109). Though important, this point does not change the basic assumption that the central capabilities are maximizable.

Is it possible to maximize the central capabilities as Roduit thinks? Unfortunately, this question defies a straightforward answer. Let me explain, why. To do that we should take a look into the central capabilities as they are described by Nussbaum. Let us start with the capability that on the Nussbaum's list usually comes first:

[9] "The ideal human that individuals are striving towards when using human enhancement should at a minimum retain the ten central capabilities; a form of human enhancement should harmoniously maximize those capabilities as a whole" (Roduit, 2016, 33).

> *Life*. Being able to live to the end of a human life of a normal length; not dying prematurely, or before one's life is so reduced as to be not worth living (Nussbaum, 2011, 33).

In what way can this capacity be enhanced or maximized? It is clear that to maximize this capability does not mean to increase the lifespan by the help of some gene editing or other biomedical technology. The capability to live life of normal length as such is not maximizable. This is just a requirement to guarantee that every individual has the capability to live a life of a normal length, given particular technological possibilities and other context-relevant circumstances.

Let us take another capability:

Bodily health. Being able to have good health, including reproductive health; to be adequately nourished; to have adequate shelter (Ibid).

This case is more interesting than the previous one. And the reason for this is that the question whether this capability is maximizable depends on how we define health. If, following Boorse (Boorse, 1977), we define health as absence of disease, then this capability turns out to be non-maximizable because if one is healthy then there is no way to get healthier than she is. However, we can derive the opposite outcome if we would choose to define health in a positive way, say, according to WHO, i.e., if we would take health to be "a state of complete physical, mental, and social well-being and not merely the absence of disease or infirmity", then the capability of health seems to be maximizable.[10] And as there are no decisive answers to the question, which definition should be preferred, there is no any straightforward way to say whether this capability is maximizable. All that we can say is – it depends.

In case of other capabilities, the situation is even less clear. For example, the capability *Senses, imagination, and thought* is described as the ability to uses senses, to imagine and to reason. On the one hand, the ability to use imagination and to reason seems to be maximizable. On the other hand, Nussbaum's qualification, that we should be able "to do these things in a "truly human" way" (Ibid.), makes the picture less clear. Moreover, from the way Nussbaum describes this capability it is clear she stresses what might be called liberty and opportunity to use the human capacities

[10] On the concept of positive health see Nordenfelt, 2017. The concept is explained and criticized in Boorse, 1977, 568–572. Ereshefsky recently suggested that medical issues should be framed in terms of state descriptions and normative claims, thus avoiding many theoretical problems that all the classical theories of health and disease tend to run into. See Ereshefsky, 2009.

in question. The same should be said about some other capabilities, such as *Emotions*, *Practical reason*, and *Affiliation*, i.e., they might be maximizable; however, from the way Nussbaum presents them, it is far from clear what it would mean to maximize them as they are described as thresholds or norms.

What I find strange in Roduit's presentation of his account is that he does not provide any details of his take on this important issue. He says, for example, that: "Maximizing the capability of emotion over practical reason or affiliation might make some individuals unable to function in society" (Roduit, 2016, 109). Unfortunately, Roduit does not elaborate on what, for example, maximizing the capability of emotion is supposed to be, as if that should be clear from Nussbaum's description. So, let us look at what Nussbaum says:

> *Emotion*. Being able to have attachments to things and people outside ourselves; to love those who love and care for us, to grieve at their absence; in general, to love, to grieve, to experience longing, gratitude, and justified anger. Not having one's emotional development blighted by fear and anxiety (Nussbaum, 2011, 33-34).

What would it mean to maximize this capability? To increase the number of things that we are able to have attachments? To increase (or decrease depending on the context and our relation to the individual we are communicating these emotions to) the intensity of those attachments? To love more or to grieve more than we normally do? Or experience more longing, gratitude, and justified anger? Some of those answers might be right and some might make no sense. My point is that from the way Nussbaum describes this capability it is far from obvious how one could maximize it (if that is possible at all). My guess is that what Nussbaum has in mind here but does not say explicitly is that all those abilities have some culture relative norms of implementation, i.e., though different cultures and different people (who have different goals and play different roles within their interpersonal relationships) might differ on this, there is something like excessive or deficient love, grief, etc. I presume that in a similar vein as in the case of the capability *Senses, imagination, and thought*, Nussbaum would add that we should able to experience those emotions in a truly human way. The only problem with this, to my mind - correct, interpretation is that this makes Roduit's account unintelligible. Again, it may be the case that Roduit has some particular idea of how the central capabilities should be interpreted, but the book and other Roduit's writings are silent on the issue. And what is even more surprising, so is Roduit's recent paper on the usefulness of his approach in the ethics of enhancement in sport (Roduit, 2017). To show the usefulness of the CA in the enhancement debate, Roduit invites us to consider the hypothetical case of Judy the boxer. To become a better boxer Judy decides to enhance herself. She finds that her compassion towards others and fears that she experiences before a competition worsens her boxing performance. So, she decides to take some sort of drug that reduces her fear and uses some mental exercises that helps her to detach herself from perceiving other people as humans. Roduit argues that from a type-perfection point of view this is not a human enhancement:

> Using the grid provided by the central capabilities, we see that Judy might put her *bodily health* at risk, but more importantly, she erodes her *emotional* capability and her capability of *affiliation*, as she might no longer be able to relate to other human beings. Thinking from a *property-perfectionist* view that she was enhancing herself, we can see that from a type-perfectionist view, she might become something other than human. She might become better at punching people, but she will not become a better *human* boxer. (Roduit, 2017, 5)

I must admit that Roduit's conclusion here strikes me as plain wrong. It seems to me that thanks to the drugs and meditation Judy in fact will become a better human boxer. There are other things that seem to me to be wrong here and I will mention at least one of them in the next section, but in the context of the present discussion the two following points are more relevant. First, the capabilities are used here only as principles that restrict enhancement and not as a guide and second, the way Roduit uses "the grid provided by the central capabilities" doesn't give any clues as to how the capabilities can be maximized.

To make things worse, there is another problem that should be mentioned here. The context of the debate is biomedical enhancement. And this means that the central capabilities should not be just maximizable (as Roduit takes them to be) but maximizable by using biomedical means. This restriction means that such capabilities as *Bodily integrity, Other species* and *Control over one's environment* should be dropped from the list as there is hardly any way how to affect them by biomedical technologies.

To conclude the discussion so far, it seems that that the idea of enhancing the central capabilities does not look promising. Some capabilities are non-maximizable and in some cases the question of the maximizability of the capability is far from clear. Moreover, some of the central capabilities cannot be affected by biomedical means. Thus, it seems that the idea that

CA can be used as a guide for human enhancement, if not hopeless, is at least deeply problematic.

Does the CA provide any incentive to enhance?

Let us change the perspective for a while and ask a different question - does CA provide any incentives for human enhancement? To answer this question, we should take a closer look at the account of the central capabilities given by Nussbaum.

The approach is designed to assess and compare societies for their decency and justice. According to CA, to do this, the key question that we should ask is - what is each person able to do and to be? As Nussbaum explains:

> The approach takes *each person as an end*, asking not just about the total or average well-being but about the opportunities available to each person. It is *focused on choice of freedom*, holding that the crucial good societies should be promoting for their people is a set of opportunities, or substantial freedoms, which people then may or may not exercise in action: the choice is theirs. It thus commits itself to respect for people's powers of self-determination. (Nussbaum, 2011, 18)

It should be clear from this passage that CA is primarily intended as a political and not anthropological theory as Roduit and others (e.g., Coeckelbergh) sometimes seem to take it.[11] It is about what one should take into account if one wants to devise a set of principles for a just and decent society that respects human worth and dignity. This is also clear from the way the concept of the central capabilities is defined. If one reads Roduit's account of CA (e.g., his description of Judy the boxer example discussed above), one may get an impression that the capabilities are actual

[11] Nussbaum is explicit that CA is not a theory about human nature: "The Capabililties Approach is not a theory of what human nature is, and it does not read norms off from innate human nature. Instead, it is evaluative and ethical from the start: it asks, among the many other things that human beings might develop the capacity to do, which ones are the really valuable ones, which are the ones that a minimally just society will endeavor to nurture and support? An account of human nature tells us what resources and possibilities we have and what our difficulties may be. It does not tell us what to value" (Nussbaum, 2011, 28).

mental or physical properties of persons that might be either enhanced or eroded. But that is a gross oversimplification of CA. The concept of the central capabilities is much more complex. Nussbaum talks about different kinds of capabilities. First, there are what she calls *basic capabilities*: innate human faculties that make later development and training possible. Then there are *internal capabilities* that Nussbaum describes as developed traits and abilities. These traits and abilities are developed in interaction with the social, economic, familial, and political environment. The central capabilities that are found in Nussbaum's list are in fact what she calls *combined capabilities* which are defined as *internal capabilities* "plus the social/political/economic conditions in which functioning can actually be chosen" (Nussbaum, 2011, 22). By describing the central capabilities as complex, Nussbaum wants to stress that they are not just abilities residing inside an individual. The capabilities are also "the freedoms or opportunities created by a combination of personal abilities and the political, social, and economic environment" (Ibid. 20). So, when Nussbaum talks, for example, about bodily health as the central capability she talks about the *ability* to have good health, i.e., about access to proper health-care, nourishment, etc. And the same applies to all other capabilities on her list. Another important distinction that Nussbaum stresses is that between capabilities and functionings (Ibid. 25). By capability she means freedom to select.[12] Functioning, on the other hand, is "active realization of one or more capabilities". To illustrate her point, she uses Sen's example of a person who is starving and a person who is fasting. As far as nutrition is concerned both have the same type of functioning, but there is difference in terms of their capability. The person who is fasting has a choice which the starving person doesn't have. CA is about promoting capabilities and not functionings. Nussbaum points out that there is huge moral difference between, on the one hand, a policy that promotes health and, one the other hand, a policy that promotes health capabilities.[13] Now it should be clear that, for example, Roduit's claim that Judy's enhancements are ruled out by CA is confused. Judy, as far as we can tell from the description of the case, has the central capabilities, she just makes (one would say, morally alarming)

[12] It is not, of course, just a random selecting. The capability responsible for proper selection is practical reason that, according to Nussbaum, together with the capability of affiliation play a distinctive architectonic role, i.e., they organize and pervade the others. See Nussbaum, 2000, 82, Nussbaum, 2011, 39.

[13] To be fair to Roduit, he is aware of the capabilities/functionings distinction (see Roduit, 2016, 106); however, when he discusses the application of the approach to human enhancement he seems to ignore it.

choices about realization of particular functionings. In that she resembles the fasting person in Sen's example.

To conclude, it seems, that the answer raised at the beginning of this section is negative. From the point of view of CA there are no incentives to use any enhancement technologies whatsoever, because CA is a political doctrine about opportunities and not functionings. If in some society people are denied some of the central capabilities, then enhancing people would not be the answer. The proper way to address that problem would be to reorganize the relevant institutions and whole society in such a way that is just and respects human dignity.

Now, one might argue that I am not fair to Roduit, that it is wrong to criticize him by pointing out that his claims don't square well with what Nussbaum says about CA. In Roduit's defense it might be said that Nussbaum's account of capabilities is tailored for a specific purpose – to assess societies for decency and justice.[14] And this is the main reason why Nussbaum concentrates on minimum thresholds, and why so much attention is paid to social aspects of capabilities in her presentation of the approach. And may be the same can be said about the problems of maximizability that were discussed before. It might be the case that in Nussbaum's account the capabilities don't allow maximization, but this is not necessarily true about Roduit's use of the approach. These seem to me fair and important points, but they still don't solve Roduit's problems. Roduit still might be right, but he owes us an account on how CA can be saved from the objections that I have raised.

Besides, from what I have said so far it does not follow that CA is useless in the human enhancement debate. In fact, there is one aspect in which our understanding of the issues around human enhancement might benefit from resources provided by CA. Many current discussions on human enhancement suffer from a certain bias towards biotechnological solutions. Especially this applies to discussions on so-called moral enhancement where some authors present moral enhancement by biomedical means as our only hope to avoid a major disaster.[15] But as de Melo-Martin and Salles (de Melo-Martin & Salles, 2015, 228) have pointed out such approach relies on a deeply suspect view that moral ills are a result of mainly individual moral deficits:

[14] I would like to thank Nick Agar for raising this issue.

[15] This view is defended by Ingmar Persson and Julian Savulescu in Persson and Savulescu 2012.

> "The framing of morally complex situations like war, famine, terrorism, lack of access to medicines, or poverty, as the result of certain types of individual moral failings ignores the role played by structural - social, cultural, political, economic - forces in enabling and often promoting these evils. In this sense, proponents of moral bioenhancement seem to entertain an oversimple conception of moral evil as abstracted from the real world."

As we just saw, Nussbaum's capabilities are combined from what she calls internal capabilities and the social, political, and economic conditions, and this means that if we think about different issues of human enhancement via the lens provided by CA, we should be more sensitive to the social determinants of human problems that human enhancement allegedly is supposed to solve.

Conclusion

The main task of this chapter is to evaluate the proposal made by Roduit that Nussbaum's capability approach can be used to assess morality of human enhancement. In the previous sections I have shown that Roduit's proposal has various problems. In particular, Roduit's claim that the capabilities approach is a type-perfectionist theory that can be used both as guiding and restricting cannot be justified. This is so for more than one reason. First, some of the central capabilities are not maximizable and for others the issue is not clear. Unfortunately, Roduit has not provided any account of the maximizability of the capabilities, but Nussbaum's account in this regard is indefinite. Second, many capabilities on Nussbaum's list are such that they cannot be affected by biomedical means. Besides, a closer examination of the capabilities approach shows that it provides no incentives for human enhancement. Of course, the capabilities approach can still be used as restricting; however, in that case one must be careful to take into account the distinction between capabilities and functionings.[16]

[16] I would like to thank the anonymous reviewer for the useful comments which helped me to improve the paper. Also, I would like to express my gratitude to Justin Caouette for checking my English and providing some useful comments about the content of the chapter.

Literature

Daniels, N. (2000) Normal Functioning and the Treatment-Enhancement Distinction, *Cambridge Quarterly of Healthcare Ethics*, 9, 309–322.

de Melo-Martini, I., Salles, A. (2015) Moral Bioenhancement: Much Ado About Nothing, *Bioethics*, 29(4), 223–232.

Boorse, Ch. (1977) Health as a Theoretical Concept, *Philosophy of Science*, 44(4), 542–573.

Buchanan, A. (2011) *Better than Human: The Promise and Perils of Enhancing Ourselves*, Oxford: Oxford University Press.

Coeckelbergh, M. (2011) Human Development or Human Enhancement? A Methodological Reflection on Capabilities and the Reevaluation of Information Technologies, *Ethics and Information Technology*, 13, 81–92.

Ereshefsky, M. (2009) Defining 'Health' and 'Disease', *Studies in History and Philosophy of Biological and Biomedical Sciences*, 40(3), 221–227.

Gyngell, C., Selgelid, M.J. (2016) Human Enhancement: Conceptual Clarity and Moral Significance, Clarke, S., Savulescu, J., Coady, C.A.J., Giubilini, A., Sanyal, S. (Eds) *The Ethics of Human Enhancement. Understanding the Debate*, Oxford: Oxford University Press, 111–126.

Harris, J. (2007) *Enhancing Evolution: The Ethical Case for Making Better People*, Princeton: Princeton University Press.

Hughes, J. (2011) After Happiness, Cyborg Virtue, *Free Inquiry*, 32(1), 1–7.

Menuz, V., Hurlimann, T., Godard, B. (2013) Is Moral Enhancement also a Personal Matter? *Science and Engineering Ethics*, 19, 161–177.

Nordenfelt, L. (2017) On Concepts of Positive Health, Schramme, T., Edwards, S. (Eds) *Handbook of the Philosophy of Medicine*, Dordrecht: Springer, 29–43.

Nussbaum, M. (1988) Nature, Function, and Capability: Aristotle on Political Distribution, *Oxford Studies in Ancient Philosophy*, Supplementary Volume I, 145–184.

Nussbaum, M. (1992) Human Functioning and Social Justice: In Defense of Aristotelian Essentialism, *Political Theory*, 20, 202–246.

Nussbaum, M. (1995) Human Capabilities, Female Human Beings, Nussbaum, M., Glover, J. (Eds) *Women, Culture and Development: A Study of Human Capabilities*, Oxford: Clarendon Press, 61–104.

Nussbaum, M. (2000) *Women and Human Development*, Cambridge: Cambridge University Press.

Nussbaum, M. (2006) *Frontiers of Justice. Disability, Nationality, Species Membership*, Cambridge and Massachusetts: Harvard University Press.

Nussbaum, M. (2011) *Creating Capabilities. The Human Development Approach*, Cambridge and Massachusetts: Harvard University Press.

Persson, I., Savulescu, J. (2012) *Unifit for the Future. The Need for Moral Enhancement*, Oxford: Oxford University Press.

Roduit, A. R. (2016) *The Case for Perfection. Ethics in the Age of Human Enhancement*, Frankfurt am Main: Peter Lang GmbH.

Roduit, J., Gaehwiler, R. (2017) Ethics and Enhancement in Sport: Becoming the Fastest (Human?) Being, *Sport in Society*, 1–7. DOI: 10.1080/17430437.2016.1273636.

Roduit, J., Heilinger, J.C., Baumann, H. (2015) Ideas of Perfection and the Ethics of Human Enhancement, *Bioethics*, 29, 622–630.

Sandel, M. (2007) *The Case against Perfection*, Cambridge and Massachusetts: The Belknap Press of Harvard University Press.

Savulescu, J. (2006) Justice, Fairness, and Enhancement, *Annals of the New York Academy of Sciences*, 1093, 321–338.

Chapter 5

The pragmatist philosophical view of human enhancement

Emil Višňovský

Abstract: The chapter provides a brief overview of the current contexts and key issues in the transhumanist idea of human enhancement. From a philosophical viewpoint transhumanism is a continuation of the ancient ideas of human perfection and perfectionism. When taken in abstracto from other ethical ideas such as happiness, dignity, self-care, and self-regulation, transhumanism may have problematic consequences. The chapter further provides an account of pragmatist philosophical humanism which suggests that at times it resembles a precursor of or a very close ally to transhumanism. However, the author concludes that, despite the fact that we can find support for the idea of 'transformism' in pragmatist humanism, ultimately it is about achieving the good life and good society, and not about the radical enhancement of biological human nature via (bio)technology.

Introduction

Contemporary transhumanism as the promotion of the idea of "human enhancement" (Bostrom, 2005; Savulescu and Bostrom, 2009) can neither be considered a straightforward anti-humanism, nor a Foucauldian or Adornian critique of humanism in the "end of man" sense or "disgust" at all that humans are capable of inflicting on one other. Rather it is "superhumanism" in the sense of improving and going beyond the natural, organic (biological) limits and potential of human beings. But what they all have in common is a rejection of human beings as we know them. Thus from the perspective of traditional humanism they can justifiably be regarded as nihilism (the annihilation of humanness). The other commonality is a concern for power – however, whilst humanism founders over power, transhumanism is built upon it.[1] Transhumanism also contains the idea of posthumanism, as R. Braidotti (2013) has pointed out, albeit from a slightly different perspective. Her view is that not even the humanism of today can simply be regarded as "positive" and unproblematic; on the contrary, it can be viewed as the root of the inhumanness we inflict upon one another, which may well be the most absurd paradox in history: crimes against humanity committed by humans in the name of a better, or rather an enhanced human race.

[1] Bostrom's latest book, *Superintelligence* (Bostrom, 2014), looks at how thanks to technology humankind is reaching a superhuman level of intelligence that will give future human beings "superpowers" over nature and over themselves.

It all comes down to what kind of being we think humans are. Transhumanists may agree with humanists (including pragmatists) that humans are beings that have ever since longed for perfection and have been endowed with a capacity for self-improvement, but they disagree on what human nature is. Humanists consider humans in their current known form, i.e. natural and cultural beings, to be the highest value, and so they wish to preserve that value. Transhumanists either have a different highest value, or they subscribe to a different conception of human nature; one that should and must be "overcome", transcended. By contrast pragmatist humanism is naturalistic, i.e. based on the natural unity between humans and the planet Earth that "gave birth" to them. Any kind of disruption to this unity would have serious consequences, whilst its preservation indicates that humans are natural earthly beings, and that there is no alternative to their natural earthly existence, no "artificial" or "cosmic" existence like that being enhanced in the minds of transhumanists.[2]

Perfectionist idea of enhancement

One can also view the current transhumanist idea of human enhancement from the perspective of perfectionism.[3] This, of course, is an ancient philosophical or ethical concept rooted in the work of Plato and Aristotle, and even in earlier mythology. In it humans adopted the idea of " becoming godlike", and this idea would persist throughout the history of culture in both religion and philosophy.[4] In Plato's dualism of the perfect world of

[2] This is not to reject exploration of the cosmos, the system to which Earth belongs, or the seeking out of opportunities to find a "second Earth" and perhaps inhabit it etc. This is the standpoint from which Elon Musk's projects can also be considered to be trans- and post-, as well as humanistic, in the sense that they proffer a visionary preservation of humanity in the future, so long as they do not completely abandon the natural part of human existence in favour of "trans-natural" artificial technology and intelligence based solely on human inventions.

[3] On distinguishing between non-humanist and humanist perfectionism and whether it applies only to humans or not, see Hurka (1996).

[4] E. Fromm (1966/1991) pointed to the cultural origins and function of the concept of God in his radical humanism. E. Gilson (1941/1994) provided an analysis of the concept of God in philosophy. L. Ferry (1996/2002) recently wrote about "transcendental" humanism and the divinization of the human. In his bestselling book Israeli historian Y. N. Harari (2014) writes about how history began with man finding God – and will end when humans become Gods, in the shape of transhuman beings.

forms and the imperfect world of things, people's ancient yearning for the transcendental and absolute were philosophically articulated in the shape of a perfectly harmonic (Pythagorean) cosmos, a perfectly unchanging (Eleatic) existence, a perfectly good moral (Socratic) life, and even a perfectly (Aristotelian) balanced human being guided by the "divine light" of reason. The idea of the perfect being is actually the idea of God, and this human desire to emulate or pursue it is a desire for immortality, a longing to eliminate deficiencies and limits, and to go beyond our natural, earthly ties. Aristotle's *eudaimonia* and the desire for a better, perfect life, inherent to human nature, is a variation on the philosophical theory of perfectionism as the theory of the greatest good, which is an end in itself, not bound to any other goal. Aristotle thought humans could achieve this by improving and developing their nature, their best features, abilities, and virtues in a moral or political sense. It was on this bedrock that the classic ideas of humanism were established as the cultivation, nurture, and development of human qualities.[5] In perfectionist humanism the meaning of human life is the striving for perfection as the highest goal, an end in itself; although clearly it is more a process than a state. Finally, there is little agreement on the criteria for, or actual form of, absolute perfection or the greatest good it should take.

Perfectionism is the antithesis of nihilism. Perfectionism which recognizes good and the perfecting of it also recognizes something that is even better than good. The fact that the desire for perfection and the idea of perfectionism (improvement) can also have a dark, negative side was not the subject of philosophical consideration until much later. For instance, in his

---

[5] Humanism is not a single intellectual and cultural movement. Subscribing to it does not therefore mean conceiving of humans, humankind, or humanness in the same way. Humanism may include an Enlightenment celebration of man, a romantic or theistic love of humans, ethical reverence for human beings, or an anthropological concern for man. The Latin etymology (*humus* - earth, soil; *homo* - earthly being; *humanus* - earthly, human) indicates that the "truly human" is most frequently posited as secular in contrast to the divine (*divinitas*), and cultural rather than natural (*animalis*), as individual or subjective in juxtaposition to social or objective. For Aristotle humans come somewhere between god and animal, and for Nietzsche humans hang above the abyss between animal and "superman" (since "God is dead"). The term has been around since Cicero, but was revived for the modern era by F. P. I. Niethammer (1766–1848) following his Renaissance *studia humanitatis*, juxtaposed with the philanthropism in his 1803 work, which led to the study of man being incorporated into universities in the Humboldtian era. Philosophically relevant conceptions, or critical interpretations of humanism, were developed by Herder (the concept of humanity), Feuerbach (*homo homini deus est*), Comte (religious humanity), Sartre, Heidegger, Adorno, Foucault, and others. Contemporary authors concerned with the issue of humanism include Soper (1986), Davis (1996), and Norman (2004).

Hegelian dialectics, Marx showed how it produces the reverse effect once a certain boundary is crossed; and Nietzsche showed how a desire for the absolute becomes a desire for power, culminating in the anti-humanism of the superhuman; whereas Freud demonstrated how the desire for the good life of the self tends to lie in the hands of the *Id* and *Super-Ego*. Instead they posited the good society (Marx), the strong individual (Nietzsche), or hedonism (Freud) as the ideal. In other words – they all drew attention to the problem of happiness, understood in different ways.

What then is the relationship between perfection and the good life or happiness? Whereas for Aristotle happiness is the highest good, Kant adopted a sceptical attitude (1793/1970) because what appears to be theoretically correct may not turn out to be correct in practice, as at least two other modern philosophers have testified on the basis of their own life experiences: J. S. Mill (1873) and W. James (James 1920). Both had to overcome intellectual and personal crises that were the outcome of being raised in a perfectionist manner by their fathers.

The theory of perfectionism, whilst appearing to be a positive and incontestable ideal, can be challenged by asking a philosophical question about its meaning. This requires it to be investigated in relation to other ethical theories: 1. the theory of happiness; 2. the theory of dignity; 3. the theory of self-care; and 4. the theory of reflective self-control. The perfectionist desire for perfection becomes problematic when it is absolutized and set against these concepts (the desire for happiness, need for dignity, self-care, and self-control).[6]

Transhumanist perfectionism

Philosophically there is nothing new or incomprehensible about transhumanist perfectionism. But its adherents have at least one additional powerful argument: not only can we enhance ourselves; indeed we must – because we have recently developed the unprecedented technologies to do so. The time has already come, so they say, for us to combine our lifelong desires or utopias with the technologies to make our ancient dreams come true and transform ourselves from earthly natural creatures into

[6] Such an investigation, however, is not the part of this chapter.

something else.[7] Social engineering is being replaced with biotechnological engineering, and this latter will provide us with unimagined and limitless opportunities for a better life (and happiness it would seem) based on science.

The prospects promised by transhumanist perfectionism look truly magnificent, if not fantastical. For instance, the British philosopher David Pearce[8] proffers a vision in which all human suffering is eliminated. He has elaborated a concept of "abolitionism", inspired by J. Bentham, that is an updated version of the utilitarian calculus for maximizing pleasure and minimizing suffering. Pearce believes that not only are there persuasive ethical reasons for having such a goal, but the technological means (genetic engineering, nanotechnologies, etc.) for achieving it also exist. His project, designed to achieve this, is called "paradise engineering" (Pearce, 1995). It will contain all living creatures (including animals) and their entire ecosystem. Like R. Rorty, who claimed that human cruelty towards other humans was not inevitable but brought about by social conditions, Pearce claims that the suffering of living creatures and humans is avoidable; the evolution of humans and life are purportedly heading towards the elimination of both physical (*via* neurosurgery) and mental suffering (*via* neuropharmacology). The use of chemical substances and drugs to alter moods and emotional states (e.g. depression) will give way to more perfect genetic engineering and nanotechnologies capable of "reprogramming" the animal essence of living creatures as predators including humans. It is also possible to use biotechnologies to treat ageing and some lifestyle diseases, such as drug addiction.

Pearce is also a proponent of the idea of "bio-happiness", expanded on in greater detail by Canadian philosopher and ethicist Mark Alan Walker. He believes that human happiness is biological in essence and can be biochemically altered by using "happiness pills" to increase potential feelings of happiness and spiritual contentment. He sees this as an ethical imperative (Walker 2013). This involves enhancing our subjective capacity for hap-

[7] The idea of transhumanism as the self-transcendence of humankind as a natural species had already been considered by Julian Huxley (1957). It is currently most radically dealt with by Ray Kurzweil (2005) in his theory of singularity; in 2008 he founded Singularity University (singularityu.org) in California. The term "singularity" was first developed in 1958 by the mathematician J. von Neumann. It was elaborated in a transhumanist sense by another mathematician, Vernon Vince (1993). There is now a wide range of authors working on the "singularity hypothesis" (Eden, Steinhart, Pearce, and Moor, 2012).

[8] D. Pearce and N. Bostrom founded the World Transhumanist Association (1998), now known as Humanity+. Their ideas and work can mainly be found on internet sites (www.lifeboat.com, www.bltc.com, www.hedweb.com).

piness or ability to feel happy, starting with the genetic manipulation of embryos through to the use of pharmacological substances.[9]

Amongst the proponents of transhuman enhancement one can also find more moderate theorists alongside the radicals. One such moderate is sociologist and bioethicist James J. Hughes, who came up with the concept of "democratic transhumanism". His concern is that perfectionist technologies should be safe and available to all, and that the individual's right to self-control should be respected (Hughes, 2004).

However, transhumanist human enhancement[10] is not just motivated by a perfectionist desire for perfection. A whole series of passions are evidently at play here, ranging from a nihilistic disgust at contemporary humanity and an obsession with scientific and technological progress to a more or less hidden desire for global world domination. This "desire for control" (dominion, rule), which may hide a quite prosaic and very "basal" desire for profit, has been critically highlighted by M. Sandel (2004). Further criticism of what modern (capitalist) society is doing to human desires and the emotional core of human nature has been expressed by many writers from Nietzsche, Marx, and Freud to Foucault, from Deleuze and Guattari to Žižek, Agamben, Stiegler, and others.

In addition to the underlying motivations and reasons for human enhancement, the consequences, whether predictable or unpredictable, are no less deserving of criticism. In some cases it is possible to know which are safe and which are risky, and in others one cannot be at all certain as to what they will bring. As philosophers from Hegel to Sartre have known, the counterfinality of human action, i.e. its unintended and unwanted effects, is the ontological side, so attempts at predicting, or at least not ignoring them, is a fundamental part of human and philosophical wisdom, which the classic pragmatists from Peirce to Dewey very well knew.[11]

---

[9] There are those who have voiced criticism of the concept of biohappiness, such as bioethicist Leon Kass (2003).

[10] Transhumanists distinguish between two basic types of enhancement: medical and non-medical (Savulescu and Bostrom, 2009).

[11] It is not only transhumanism but the entire global obsession with technological and scientific progress and the potentialities involved that have attracted radical criticism. Bill McKibben (1989; 2004), for example, points to the negative and unacceptable side of human interference in nature, from the ecological to the existential consequences. The "existential risks" presented by scientific and technological development today and the possibility it may lead to human extinction are the subject of multidisciplinary analyses by the Centre for the Study of Existential Risk in Cambridge, England (http://cser.org).

Pragmatist humanism

All humanisms are humanisms because they consider the good of a person to be the highest value, since all humanisms contain within them the idea of enhancing (refining) humans or their lives and conditions. This need not be anthropocentrism in a "humans are the centre of the universe" sense, but rather that humans are the "centre of their human world". From this perspective then pragmatist humanism should not have a problem with transhumanism or with the idea of human enhancement. However, it is more complicated than this.

Humanism was first introduced into the debate on classic pragmatism by F. C. S. Schiller.[12] He called it "epistemic humanism", since he was concerned with the concepts of knowledge and truth, which are human creations and expressions of specific human interests.[13] He openly defended anti-sceptical relativism. He thought one could never overlook human needs and desires, and in this there is an echo of Nietzsche's *menschliches, allzumenschliches* despite Nietzsche being the grandfather of modern anti-humanism. Schiller's philosophy is a radical apology for subjectivity and as such criticizes traditional logic for being a dehumanized human concern that is nothing other than a tool for satisfying human goals.[14] He thought humanism was a better, more general, name for the philosophy than pragmatism, but a true humanist must also be a pragmatist, since he cannot escape into abstraction and lose contact with reality. He defined humanism as the "systematic protest against the artificial elimination of

[12] Ferdinand Canning Scott Schiller (1864–1937) was an Oxford philosopher and logician, a British critic of the British Hegelians (F. H. Bradley) and the analytics (B. Russell), and the main classic pragmatist theorist in Europe. He had independently produced his own version of pragmatism, which he called "humanism", by the time he had completed his first work, the *Riddles of the Sphinx* (1891). On his first trip to the USA he encountered W. James and his work at Cornell University (1893–1897). The two philosophers communicated at length and were of mutual inspiration to one another. Schiller was considered to be a "modern Protagoras", defending his *homo-mensura*, a concept he explored most in an article entitled "Axioms as Postulates" (1902) and in his books *Humanism* (1903) and *Studies in Humanism* (1907). He was made a professor at Oxford, and from 1926 onwards lived and lectured at universities in California, where he would die.

[13] Many have discussed the conditionality between knowledge and interests: Hegel, Marx, even Habermas; however, whilst they were more concerned with social and group interests, Schiller had only individual interests in mind.

[14] J. Dewey systematically elaborated pragmatist logic in this spirit. C. S. Peirce may have expressed respect for Schiller's humanism, but both he and Dewey rejected Schiller's concept of logic.

the human aspects of knowing in the intellectualist versions of logic and psychology" (Schiller, 1924/2008, 93). Humanism for him is "the simplest of philosophical standpoints" expressing the "perception that the philosophic problem concerns human being striving to comprehend a world of human experience by the resources of human minds" (Schiller, 1912/2008, 52). However, his humanism is both epistemological and metaphysical:

> Humanism has no quarrel with the assumptions of common-sense realism; it does not deny what is popularly described as the 'external' world. It has far too much respect for the pragmatic value of conceptions which de facto work far better than those of the metaphysics which despise and try to supersede them. It insists only that the 'external world' of realism is still dependent on human experience, and perhaps ventures to add also that the data of human experience are not completely used up in the construction of a real external world (Schiller, 1912/2008, 52–53).

External reality is flexible and can be shaped by human beings in their image; it is anthropomorphic. Humans not only shape truth but also reality itself; nothing is absolutely given without there being a subjective contribution, benefit, or sharing.

Schiller applied this general philosophical conception to an area that is particularly interesting in relation to human enhancement. That subject was eugenics, something he studied systematically for many years.[15] He argued in favour of eugenics, which he saw as the future and saviour of humanity, almost making him the forerunner of the transhumanists. He considered human nature to be a set of potentialities that could be improved. Eugenics contains the idea that there are ideal human characteristics around which society should be organized; e.g. it is bad if the most talented people do not have children. Eugenics set out moral ideals for progressive and reformist social aims. Schiller backed the national "family improvement" programme, but rejected racism and fascism. He drew a distinction on the one hand between "negative eugenics" as a method of protecting against human and social collapse, and "positive eugenics" on the other as a way to "*improve* the human race and to lift human life to a higher level" (Schiller, 1932/2008, 367–368).

[15] Schiller was founding member, vice-president, and member of the governing board of the English Eugenics Society (1907). He wrote three books on the subject: *Tantalus or the Future of Man* (1924), *Eugenics and Politics* (1926), and *Social Decay and Eugenic Reform* (1932). For more details see Skodo (2015).

Although Schiller explicitly viewed his eugenics papers as applications of humanism, rather than pragmatism (although for him the two were identical), his philosophy was directly inspired by the Italian branch of "magic pragmatism" as promoted by Giovanni Papini and Giuseppe Prezzolini.[16] He discovered this philosophy through Benedetto Croce, whose aesthetics were a celebration of limitless human creativity. They rejected rationality as the main human quality and consequently also intellectualism and positivism. Philosophy, thought Papini, should become "active, creative, taking its part in a necessary reformation of the world"; and that philosophy was pragmatism, a "philosophy of act, philosophy of action, reconstruction, transformation, creation!" (Papini, 1924, 119; 204). For them pragmatism was a philosophical programme that would enable man to become "a rival of Divinity", to transform himself from a "poor, week, miserable creature" into a "supreme and sovereign creature, absolutely exuberant and mighty" (Papini, 1924, 130; 207). Papini later resigned himself to the "wild era" of quasi-pragmatist megalomania that brought him closer to Mussolini,[17] and converted to Catholicism (1921), whilst Prezzolini wrote in radical defence of the James-Schiller conception in conversation with G. Vailatti and M. Calderoni, proponents of the other, Peircean, branch of pragmatism in Italy.[18] He wrote articles about "L'Uomo Dio" and about his ability to change everything and shape it in accordance with his will and imagination. This voluntaristic pragmatism can also been seen as the precursor to transhumanism.

Schiller's humanism was picked up directly by William James, although his understanding of the relationship between pragmatism and humanism is quite different: humanism is just one part of pragmatism. Pragmatism is therefore a humanist philosophy in the sense that "[i]n many familiar objects every one will recognize the human element. We conceive a given reality in this way or in that, to suit our purpose, and the reality passively submits to the conception" (James, 1907/1921, 251). This "humanistic principle" means

---

[16] Giovanni Papini (1881–1956) and Giuseppe Prezzolini (1882–1982) were Italian journalists and writers, who founded the periodical and radical intellectual movement around the journal *Leonardo* (1903–1907), and who took inspiration from W. James's philosophy during his visits to Florence (1905).

[17] In an interview in 1926 B. Mussolini even boasted that "[T]he pragmatism of William James was of great use to me in my political career", because it taught him that "an action should be judged rather by its results" and so it is to "that faith in action" that "Fascism owes a great part of its success..." (quoted in Myers 1986, 414).

[18] Giovanni Vailati (1862–1909) and Mario Calderoni (1879–1914) were Italian philosophers of science, inspired primarily by Peirce's logic and semiotics, who founded a school that still continues in Italy today.

> you can't weed out the human contribution. Our nouns and adjectives are all humanized heirlooms, and in the theories we build them into, the inner order and arrangement is wholly dictated by human considerations, intellectual consistency being one of them. Mathematics and logic themselves are fermenting with human rearrangements; physics, astronomy and biology follow massive cues of preference (James, 1907/1921, 254–255).

James's pragmatist humanism is expressed in his theory of truth, and here he agreed with Schiller that to an "unascertainable extent our truths are man-made products too" (James, 1907/1921, 242). This could also be seen in his ethics and philosophical beliefs. Both were linked by the "doctrine of meliorism... Meliorism treats salvation as neither inevitable nor impossible. It treats it as a possibility, which becomes more and more of a probability the more numerous the actual conditions of salvation become" (James, 1907/1921, 286). However, the idea that occupies centre place in James's ethics is the concept of life and its value to humans. For James life is open - part of an open pluralist universe - containing uncertainty and risk, in which there is an absence of absolute rules and guidelines on the good and on the need to continually adapt to the changing circumstances, i.e. being possessed with a "strenuous belief", which involves continual effort and the active pursuit and creation of good. On the one hand a moral life means tolerance for plural forms, and reverence and respect for others, whilst on the other it means not succumbing to "fate's" obstacles and difficulties. Only an active life is one worth living and even though there are no rational arguments for meliorism - i.e. for improving life - or any kind of guarantee, emotional forces exist that will continually guide us towards it. One such force is the "will to believe", and faith that the world can be improved.

James's philosophy and ethics does not specify in any way what this improved world might mean. He leaves it as an open project because he believes in the creativity of human's passionate nature. He does not believe in the perfect life, but he does believe that we should strive to achieve something higher that extends beyond the person. That thing, which can extend beyond a natural, mortal human being, is the possibility that there might exist another, richer "kingdom" of life, God or immortality. It was clear to him that no such thing had ever been theoretically or scientifically proven, but he was intrigued by the way it acted as a practical life force (James, 1930).

John Dewey became an advocate of humanism when he signed the *Humanist Manifesto* in 1933;[19] however, unlike James he rejected Schil-

[19] This was the first in a series of American humanist manifestos signed by many intellectu-

ler's subjectivist conception, preferring to see humanism as an aspect of his naturalism, through which he protested against the uprooting of the human (anthropological) side from nature, the separation of the human race from nature, and the dualistic view of culture and nature. In his main ontological treatise *Experience and Nature* he stated that his philosophy could also be called "naturalistic humanism" (Dewey, 1925, 10). However, he viewed the term "humanism" with great reservation because he had no use for the deification of human ("a humanistic religion"). He later used the term "anthro-inflation" to reject anthropocentrism (Dewey, 1935/1987, 85).

Dewey's humanism is inevitably bound up with his theory of democracy, so one can justifiably call it "democratic humanism" (Rockefeller, 1991). It is a kind of "social perfectionism" in which the role of the state is to positively "promote or cultivate among citizens the dispositions, habits, and virtues requisite to human flourishing" unlike the "neutralists" who only wish to protect the citizen's right to life, liberty, property, and happiness (Talisse and Aikin, 2008, 134). But herein lies the problem, a contradiction in fact, because, since Dewey's concept of democracy includes a plurality of values and ways of life, it cannot favour one concept of human flourishing over another, but has to leave this choice up to the individual (Talisse and Aikin, 2008, 135–137).

One can agree with this, since the problem concerns Dewey's concept of "growth". It is his equivalent term for "improvement". In his article titled "What humanism means to me", Dewey wrote: "What Humanism means to me is an expansion, not a contraction, of human life, an expansion in which nature and the science of nature are made the willing servants of human good" (Dewey, 1930/1984, 267). For him "growth" is the "only moral end" (Dewey, 1920/1982, 181); the natural side of every human experience, qualitative rather than quantative; the cultivation, enrichment, appreciation, deepening, improvement, and fulfilment of life, not just its expansion. He did not see growth as a fixed end in itself but as a continual process that could be another feature of the approaching transhumanism. Growth is the "ability of human experience to generate the aims and methods by which further experience shall grow in ordered richness..."; it is to "open the road and point the way to new and better experiences" (Dewey, 1939/2001, 645). For Dewey, growth is the equivalent of Aristotle's *eudaimonia*.

---

als, academics, and other thinkers, even public officials, regardless of religious, political, or philosophical persuasion. One of the authors of the second manifesto from 1973 was the pragmatist humanist P. Kurtz (1925–2012). The third manifesto (2003) was published by the American Humanist Association and signed by 21 Nobel Prize winners.

Dewey considered education to be the main sphere for human growth, development, or improvement. He thought the main purpose of schools was to develop social skills and better connections with life (Dewey, 1899)

> Since growth is the characteristic of life, education is all one with growing; it has no end beyond itself. The criterion of the value of school education is the extent in which it creates a desire for continued growth and supplies means for making the desire effective in fact (Dewey, 1916/1930, 62).

In education growth is a process of transitioning from immaturity, powerlessness, dependency, and lack of self-sufficiency to their polar opposites, by means of learning habits (Dewey, 1916/1930, 49–59). Dewey made this distinction: growth is improvement but it does not mean progressing towards a fixed idea of perfection (Dewey, 1916/1930, 65–79).

Another person who was not keen on "-isms" was Richard Rorty, whose attitude to humanism was one of ambivalence. Indeed K. Soper pondered over whether Rorty was a humanist or an anti-humanist (Soper, 2001, 115–129). Her analysis indicates quite clearly that he was a humanist, and in several ways: 1. as an anti-theist who rejected the idea that the human race was dependent on a non-human force; 2. as a Promethean anthropocentrist who celebrates the freedom and self-confidence with which the human race controls its destiny; 3. as a meliorist who believes in human progress. But Rorty is also an anti-humanist insofar as he rejects a teleological view of human history. Soper was not entirely clear on whether Rorty, despite some of his statements, did not recognize a universal human nature or whether he was in full agreement with Sartre that human was a being "destined" for self-creation. Rorty's answer to this was: "I am a humanist in the first two senses, but not in the third. I have no faith in human benevolence, though I have hopes for it" (Rorty, 2001, 133). He considered himself to be a realist and an essentialist, in that his conception of human recognized universal features that humans share with other animals and nature, and also with other people; in the first instance these are biological features, and in the second the ability to create and use language. He ascribed an important role to self-creation but did not consequently consider humans to be almighty beings, and he certainly saw no reason for them to be obsessed with their own power.

Rorty was, however, quite clearly considered a humanist by many of those who interpreted his work (Kolenda, 1990; Bernstein, 2010). Bernstein thought Rorty's humanism was "a deep and persistent humanism that is characteristic of his life and thinking" and that it consisted in his strong belief, as well as in the dominant theme of his philosophizing, that "[t]here *is nothing that we can rely on but ourselves and our fellow human beings*" (Bernstein, 2010, 201, 211). For Rorty human beings only have responsibility to one another and not to a non-human entity. His whole philosophy was motivated out of a concern for human beings, out of a feeling of empathy, sympathy, and solidarity, out of the hope of removing injustices, humiliation, and pointless cruelty, and it was an attempt to rise above all of these. Nonetheless, in the later years of his life he had serious concerns about its future:

> If I had to bet, I would bet that within a few centuries we shall have reverted to post-nuclear holocaust barbarism, and that all the good work done by the Enlightenment and by Romanticism will have to be done again. But 1 do not think such a reversion is inevitable, any more than I think that continuous progress is inevitable (Rorty, 2001, 133).

Conclusion

Pragmatist humanism is a humanism

> that requires that philosophical and scientific work be extensions of and relevant to the values and purposes of human lives. The objects of concern for our theoretical enterprises are those of improving our lives and of safeguarding what is valuable, and of opening new possibilities. Philosophical reflection that spurns the human significance of its findings is worthless theorizing (Talisse and Aikin, 2008, 86).

It is a view that holds that human problems,

> whether they be personal, social, political, environmental, or any other sort, are of our own making or are simply consequences of the circumstances we find ourselves in and that the problems are ours to solve. Furthermore, the principles on which we act, or on which we say we should act are themselves of our own making (Ryder, 2013, 288).

It is a humanism that is naturalistic and secular because it turns to the human race itself, which has no one else to rely on (Rorty, 1998, 127; Rorty,

2007, 134). Other strands of this kind of humanism are fallibilism and experimentalism: "As every scientist knows, in any particular case we might be wrong, and we must therefore be prepared to revise our ideas, our principles, and our actions according to the adequacy of their consequences" (Ryder, 2013, 293). Pragmatist humanism has no final, single correct answer to all our problems, but it does allow us to "apply creative and experimental methods to the problems we face" (Ryder, 2013, 293).

The pragmatist view of the enhancement of humans and human life is both naturalistic and humanistic, and this, despite its "transformist" character, means that whilst it promotes the idea of change, development, and growth, it has nothing to say about radical interventions to mankind's biological and existential conditions or to human nature as known throughout human history. It has nothing to say about the use of technology to overcome our biological essence.[20] It suggests we view human enhancement in terms of what it means for the good life, the happiness of the individual, and the good of society, whilst recognizing the value of pluralism, which cannot be used to decide in advance whether or what type of enhancement is good nor who it is good for. Nonetheless, Peirce's pragmatic maxim is one way of prudently ascertaining this (Višňovský, 2015). Even some transhumanists say that any loss of humanness risks a dangerous self-destructive excursion into the unknown (Agar, 2010). Thus despite pragmatism being a "philosophy of transformation" advocating "meliorism" in every way of human life, it would be a great simplification to equate it with the philosophical grounding of contemporary transhumanism. There is no such thing as a "pragmatist transhumanism" in the philosophical sense of a term (at least up to date). Pragmatism is a kind of humanism and its relation to transhumanist strategies of human enhancement requires more work to be done in the near future.

Acknowledgement

This work was supported by Slovak Research and Development Agency contract No. APVV-0379-12.

[20] Other aspects need to be explored through the pragmatist philosophy of technology and pragmatist bioethics, but that is beyond the reach of this chapter.

Literature

Agar, N. (2010) *Humanity's End. Why We Should Reject Radical Enhancement*, Cambridge, Massachusetts and London: A Bradford Book.

Bernstein, R. (2010) *The Pragmatic Turn*, Cambridge: Polity.

Bostrom, N. (2005) A History of Transhumanist Thought, *Journal of Evolution and Technology* 14, 1-25.

Bostrom, N. (2006) A Short History of Transhumanist Thought, *Analysis and Metaphysics* 5, 63-95.

Bostrom, N. (2014) *Superintelligence: Paths, Dangers, Strategies*, Oxford: Oxford University Press.

Braidotii, R. (2013) *Posthumanism*, Cambridge: Polity Press.

Davis, T. (1996) *Humanism*, London and New York: Routledge.

Dewey, J. (1899) *School and Society*, Chicago: The University of Chicago Press.

Dewey, J. (1916/1930) *Democracy and Education*, New York: The Macmillan Company.

Dewey, J. (1920/1982) *Reconstruction in Philosophy*, in *The Middle Works of John Dewey, Volume 12, 1899-1924*, Carbondale and Edwardsville: Southern Illinois University Press, 77-203.

Dewey, J. (1925/1981) *Experience and Nature*, in *The Later Works of John Dewey, Volume 5, 1929-1930*, Carbondale and Edwardsville: Southern Illinois University Press.

Dewey, J. (1930/1984) What Humanism Means to Me, in *The Later Works of John Dewey, Volume 5, 1929-1930*, Carbondale and Edwardsville: Southern Illinois University Press, 263-266.

Dewey, J. (1935/1987) Mystical Naturalism and Religious Humanism, in *The Later Works of John Dewey, Volume 11, 1935-1937*, Carbondale and Edwardsville: Southern Illinois University Press, 84-85.

Dewey, J. (1939/1988) Creative Democracy—The Task Before Us, in *The Later Works of John Dewey, Volume 14, 1939-1941*, Carbondale and Edwardsville: Southern Illinois University Press, 224-230.

Eden, A. H., Steinhart, E., Pearce, D., and Moor, J. H. (Eds) (2012) *Singularity Hypotheses*, Berlin and Heidelberg: Springer-Verlag.

Ferry, L. (1996/2002) *Man Made God: The Meaning of Life*, Chicago: The University of Chicago Press.

Fromm, E. (1966/1991) *You Shall Be as Gods*, New York: Henry Holt & Co.

Gilson, E. (1941/2002) *God and Philosophy*, New Haven and London: Yale University Press.

Harari, Y. N. (2014) *Sapiens:* A Brief History of Humankind, London: Harvill Secker.

Hughes, J. J. (2004) *Citizen Cyborg: Why Democratic Societies Must Respond to the Redesigned Human of the Future*, Boulder/Colorado: Westview Press.

Hurka, T. (1996) *Perfectionism*, Oxford: Oxford University Press.

Huxley, J. (1957) *New Bottles for New Wine*, London: Chatto & Windus.

James, W. (1902) *Varieties of Religious Experience*, New York: Longmans, Green, and Co.

James, W. (1907/1921) *Pragmatism*, New York: Longmans, Green, and Co.

James, H. (Ed) (1920) *The Letters of William James*, Boston: The Monthly Atlantic Press.

Kant, I. (1793/1970) On the Common Saying: This May Be True in Theory, but It Does Not Apply in Practice, in Reiss, H. (Ed) *Kant's Political Writings*, Cambridge: Cambridge University Press, 61–92.

Kass, L. (2003) The Pursuit of Biohappiness, *Washington Post*, October 16, available online: http://www.aei.org/article. Accessed on 03. 06. 2018.

Kolenda, K. (1990) *Rorty's Humanistic Pragmatism: Philosophy Democratized*, Tampa: University of South Florida Press.

Kurzweil, R. (2005) *The Singularity Is Near: When Humans Transcend Biology*, New York: Viking.

McKibben, B. (1989) *The End of Nature*, New York: Random House.

McKibben, B. (2004) *Enough: Staying Human in an Engineered Age*, New York: Holt.

Mill, J. S. (1873) *The Autobiography of John Stuart Mill*, London: Longmans.

Myers, G. E. (1986) *William James. His Life and Thought*, New Haven and London: Yale University Press.

Norman, R. (2004) *On Humanism*, London and New York: Routledge.

Papini, G. (1924) *The Failure*, New York: Harcourt, Brace and Company.

Pearce, D. (1995) *The Hedonistic Imperative*, available online: https://cl.nfshost.com/david-pearce-the-hedonistic-imperative.pdf. Accessed on 03. 06. 2018.

Rockefeller, S. C. (1991) *John Dewey: Religious Faith and Democratic Humanism*, New York: Columbia University Press.

Rorty, R. (1998) *Truth and Progress. Philosophical Papers, vol. 3*, Cambridge: Cambridge University Press.

Rorty, R. (2001) Response to Kate Soper, in Festenstein, M., Thompson, S. (Eds) *Richard Rorty: Critical Dialogues*, Cambridge: Polity, 130–133.

Rorty, R. (2007) *Philosophy as Cultural Politics. Philosophical Papers, vol. 4*, Cambridge: Cambridge University Press.

Ryder, J. (2013) *The Things in Heaven and Earth*, New York: Fordham University Press.

Sandel, M. (2004) The Case against Perfection, *Atlantic Monthly*, 293, 3, 51–62.

Savulescu, J., and Bostrom, N. (Eds) (2009) *Human Enhancement*, Oxford: Oxford University Press.

Schiller, F. C. S. (1912/2008) Studies in Humanism, in Shook, J. R., Macdonald, H. P. (Eds) *F. C. S. Schiller on Pragmatism and Humanism*, Amherst, NY: Humanity Books, 45–60. Schiller, F. C. S. (1924/2008) Why Humanism? in Shook, J. R., Macdonald, H. P. (Eds) *F. C. S. Schiller on Pragmatism and Humanism*, Amherst, NY: Humanity Books, 87–105.

Schiller, F. C. S. (1932/2008): Eugenics as a Moral Ideal, in Shook, J. R., Macdonald, H. P. (Eds) *F. C. S. Schiller on Pragmatism and Humanism*, Amherst, NY: Humanity Books, 367–377.

Skodo, A. (2015) Eugenics and Pragmatism: F. C. S. Schiller's Philosophical Politics, *Modern Intellectual History* 12, 1–27.

Soper, K. (1986) *Humanism and Anti-Humanism*, London: Hutchinson.

Soper, K. (2001) Richard Rorty: Humanist and/or Anti-humanist? in Festenstein, M., Thompson, S. (Eds) *Richard Rorty: Critical Dialogues*, Cambridge: Polity, 115–129.

Talisse, R. B., and Aikin, S. F. (2008) *Pragmatism. A Guide for the Perplexed*, London: Continuum.

Vince, V. (1993) The Coming Technological Singularity: How to Survive in the Post-Human Era, available online: http://www.aleph.se/Trans/Global/Singularity/sing.html. Accessed on 03. 06. 2018.

Višňovský, E. (2015) Peirce and/or Rorty? (Two Versions of Pragmatism: An Attempt at their Creative Reconciliation), in Derajová, M., Mihina, F. (Eds), *Charles Sanders Peirce: From the Philosopher's Heritage*, Bratislava: IRIS, 33–46.

Walker, M. A. (2013) *Happy-People-Pills For All*, Oxford: Wiley–Blackwell.

Chapter 6

Relevance of ontological and anthropological concepts in synthetic biology

Jana Tomašovičová

Abstract: Synthetic biology is a new research area in which the goal is to create new lifeforms. This raises a number of important questions in philosophy. In this chapter the author begins by outlining the basic research strategies used in synthetic biology and then goes on to explore the associated ontological and anthropological problems. At the ontological level, she reflects on the criteria for determining the ontological status of a synthetically created organism and on the criteria for distinguishing between complex biological systems and artefacts. Despite being synthetic in origin the resulting organism will display properties and developmental processes found in complex living organisms, consequently the author argues in favour of an ontological interpretation in which these organisms are conceived of as wholes, as is the case in ontological interpretations of natural living organisms. At the anthropological level she considers the extent to which new knowledge in synthetic biology is changing the human image and self-understanding. Since both life and human beings are viewed as having been constituted culturally and historically within a scientific framework, and given the relatively stable as well as currently changing forms of knowledge, it is important to reflect on what the consequences of new knowledge might be for the anthropological conception of human beings.

Introduction[1]

Decoding the genome has opened up new perspectives in biological research. This means that it is now possible in biology to access the molecular level of living organisms, expand existing knowledge and pave the way for new research and experimental projects. Biology had traditionally been concerned with describing and analysing existing lifeforms, but interest shifted towards the possibility that organisms could be deliberately modified and entirely new complex biological systems built. Thus a new research area known as synthetic biology emerged. This differs from classical gene technologies, also increasingly used in the modification and optimization of basic life processes, in that it is not just about altering individual genes or short gene sequences within an existing organism. In synthetic biology attempts are being made to create complex biological systems with

[1] The text is a revised version of the study Tomašovičová, J. (2018) Nové formy života? Filozofické reflexie syntetickej biológie [New Forms of Life? Philosophical Reflections on Synthetic Biology].

new properties and functions that have thus far not been found in nature (Billerbeck and Panke 2012, 20). It relies on knowledge from various scientific and technological disciplines. And is closely linked to the extensive analytic knowledge on molecular and cell biology, biochemistry and the rapidly developing knowledge in the technological and information sciences. A specific example of this is converging science, in which various technological approaches are brought together and combined, and where the research focus is on the interface between the natural and artificial spheres (Eichinger 2011, 77).

As with almost any new research area synthetic biology raises a number of questions that pose a challenge to philosophical thinking. In this chapter we will first outline the basic research strategies in synthetic biology and then explore the associated ontological and anthropological problems of this new research area. The controversy in ontological research mainly concerns the ontological status of synthetically created organisms. Should they be considered artefacts because they are created by chemical synthesis or living organisms if we take into account all their resultant properties and behaviours? In what way are complex living organisms ontologically different from artefacts? On the anthropological level we will look at an intensely debated issue, namely the extent to which new synthetic biological knowledge has an effect on changes to the anthropological human image and its self-understanding. Synthetic biology has great hidden potential to create new forms of life from scratch and so naturally raises many more relevant questions, whether they be in the ethical or environmental spheres.

1. Research approaches in synthetic biology

It is not easy to create synthetic systems - even very basic ones - that are viable, i.e. have the ability to grow, multiply, take in and convert energy and evolve. A number of experimental approaches are being used in synthetic biology to attempt to achieve this (Boldt, Müller and Maio 2009, 21–25). One is the *top-down* method, in which minimal cells are created to serve as the motherboard (the chassis) for the transplantation of synthetically created genes, or gene sequences. One way of creating this motherboard is to minimize the genome of the existing microorganism such that it only has the basic properties essential to life. However, this assumes that we are able to identify a minimal set of genes required to sustain basic life processes and that we have the methods of achieving this (Billerbeck and Panke 2012, 31; Bölker 2011, 33). In 1995 a research team at the Craig Venter Institute succeeded in decoding the genome of the *Mycoplasma genitalium* bacterium and reduced several genes to create minimal cells (Venter et al. 1995, 397–403).

This is closely related to genome synthesis, which is another research goal in synthetic biology. In natural biological systems heritable information is copied, but it is now possible to create long DNA sequences using chemical synthesis. This makes it possible to introduce an entirely new design into the genome, which could be proposed on the basis of need. However, to do so successfully would depend on a number of factors. These range from the need to understand the close connections between the various genes and the desired properties of the cells to the ability to accurately synthesize long DNA sequences using gene technologies, independently of their natural template (Billerbeck and Panke 2012, 32). In 2010 J. Craig Venter's team chemically synthesized the complete genome of the *Mycoplasma mycoides* bacterium, which was then transplanted into the specially prepared cell bacterium, *Mycoplasma capricolum*. The emergent synthesized cell was viable and continued to develop as the *M. mycoides* bacterium (Gibson et al. 2010, 52–56). However, we should note that this synthesized genome was still just a copy of the natural genome of the bacterium, the only change being the insertion of a watermark (a code containing the Venter team's contact details). It is therefore still too early to talk about the synthesis of an artificial genome in the true sense; nonetheless, the first steps to achieving this have been taken (Achatz 2013, 48).

Synthetic biology draws together knowledge from different scientific disciplines and so various specific research ambitions have emerged within it. These include the attempt to create new models and simulations of important life processes using computer technologies, known as *in silico* (Deplazes-Zemp 2011, 97). Other research goals include the creation of a synthetic protocell, which would gradually display signs of life. This would mean creating a new living organism from basic building blocks (*the bottom-up approach*). Synthetic biology is increasingly popular amongst the younger generation of scientists and students who have the opportunity through iGEM, an international competition, to design and modify some of the properties of natural lifeforms. The new genetic models are stored in a databank and can be used to build a variety of experimental constructions thanks to the existence of an assembly standard (BioBricks) (Boldt, Müller and Maio 2009, 37–38). In synthetic biology these synthetic creations are an important knowledge tool and strategy for dealing with the enormous complexity of biological systems. Once a biological system, composed of multiple components, including newly-created synthetic ones, "runs like a machine, each component can then be allocated a function that can be used to gain a far better understanding of how the molecules involved work". (Reth 2012, 45) Biologist Michael Reth suggests that the axiom, "*What I cannot create, I do not understand*", developed by atomic physicist Richard Feynman, applies in synthetic biology (Feynman in Reth 2012, 45). Synthetic biology is about advancing knowledge in biology so that we are again one step closer to gaining a better understanding.[2]

2. Ontological status of synthetic organisms

The aim of synthetic biology to create artificial lifeforms from basic building blocks has sparked a debate on definitions of their ontological status. Synthetic systems have the characteristic properties of living organisms. However, they did not develop naturally but were built out of basic biochemical components under laboratory conditions, and this blurs the original distinction between living and non-living entities. This ambiguity is further reinforced by the terms given to the products of synthetic biology, such as "living machine" or "artificial cell", which juxtapose the living with the non-living, giving the impression that living things can be seen as artefacts or biochemical machines (Boldt 2012, 182). Hence the question is whether we can consider synthetic cells to be artefacts because of their origin and method of creation, since this latter shares similar features to the construction of artefacts, or whether we can categorize them as living organisms on account of the end quality, which is comparable to that of natural biological systems. Or do we need to think about a new ontological category that would satisfactorily capture the specific nature of the synthetic cells located at the interface between natural and artificial creations?

[2] Michael Reth considers synthetic biology to be more a tool of knowledge than a method for altering nature. In a wider sense, developments in synthetic biology have partly followed those in chemistry, which was descriptive and mainly analytical until synthetic chemistry emerged at the beginning of the twentieth century. Synthetic chemistry was historically both a method for generating new materials and an important knowledge tool. The natural sciences as one might expect adopted a similar path to biology (Reth 2012, 45).

To interpret the products of synthetic biology as artefacts requires us to identify their common features. Within ontology there is a lively debate on ontological definitions of artefacts, ranging from conceptions that attempt to eliminate artefacts from ontology to theories considering them to have the ontological status of a substance. The most interesting and relevant of these to this chapter is the positive interpretation of artefacts found in the work of George Gasser. Gasser formulated his interpretation in confrontation with eliminating conceptions (Van Inwagen; Hoffman and Rosenkrantz), according to which artefacts do not represent anything new from the ontological perspective, they are merely groups of simples ordered in a certain way. This would mean that the only ontologically relevant parts are the material parts, of which artefacts consist (Van Inwagen in Gasser 2008, 129). However, Gasser thinks that, unlike simple clusters or aggregates of simples, which generally lack a form, structure or function of some kind, artefacts have a specific form; their parts are organized in a specific way, and they have a specific function. They therefore are functional unities (*funktionale Einheit*), which means the individual parts are organized in such a way as to fulfil the function ascribed to them by the designer (Gasser 2008, 132–133). These components may have preceded the artefacts in time but ontologically the individual components are equal to the artefacts.

On this view then synthetically created cells can also be seen in the first instance as functional unities. Their building components are organized in a specific way, and this enables them to perform a certain function. The genes are organized within the genome such that they fulfil a certain role, leading the cells to behave in a particular way. Similarly, as with artefacts, the resultant behaviour of the synthetic cells is largely in the hands of the designer whose ambition is to design and synthesize a genome that corresponds to current requirements.

This line of interpretation is framed within the tradition of reductionism. Reductionism is based on the assumption that complex systems can be explained if we have knowledge of the smaller parts constituting them. Hence if we know what the basic components and their functions are, we should be able to explain phenomena observed at a higher level of the organization (Mayr 2002, 23-29). It is not a great stretch then to view the higher level of the organization as a functional unity enabled by the functioning of its various parts. Reductionism is a methodological tool that has been successfully applied in various research areas, especially physics. In biology though its position is more problematic, especially when it is seen not just as a methodological strategy in research but also as a means of more generally explaining biological phenomena. Biologists view biological systems as being highly complex and as having emerged out of the multiple interactions and mutual effects at various levels of the system, i.e. between the building blocks of the organism and also between the organism and its environment (Billerbeck and Panke 2012, 26). Even the simplest of organisms have this degree of complexity, making them both fascinating and hard to understand in their entirety. At the same time their biological parts are often multifunctional, and so accurately describing their function within the system is extremely complicated (Reth 2012, 47). Their highly complex, multifunctional and variable interactions make it difficult to understand these biological systems by merely reducing them to their simplest parts. This approach can only provide us with an incomplete explanation. Ernst Mayr suggests that if we want to look at mutual interactions in biological systems at different levels, then we have to look at the system as a whole (Mayr 2002, 23–29).

In synthetic biology, this means that where there is interaction with biological systems, including artificially created ones, having an ontological understanding of them as functional unities does not suffice. Although they emerge through chemical synthesis rather than evolution, they go on to develop as living organisms. And it is the very complexity of living organisms and the close interdependency of many of their characteristic properties, such as metabolism, reproduction, self-organization or the ability to evolve,[3] that constitute good reason for ontologically interpreting living organisms as wholes. Gasser is another who argues in favour of distinguishing between unity (*Einheit*) and whole (*Ganzheit*), thereby making it possible to describe the difference between an artefact and a living organism. He holds that unlike artefacts, which are composed of individual components, wholes do not truly consist of parts that would have existed before the whole came into being. In the case of a whole, parts are rather results of a later scientific research and of natural-scientific processes of division. The parts of a living organism are not individual ontological units in their own right and so, from the ontological perspective, living organisms can be seen first and foremost as wholes (Gasser 2008, 140–142). Peter Sýkora makes a similar argument when he states: "It's not that it [the whole] could not be divided into its parts, but the existence of the parts cannot be explained without the understanding and existence of the whole that they constitute". (Sýkora 2008,

[3] Although there is still debate about the descriptions of all the characteristic properties of living organisms, 'at least three properties must exist at the biological level before we can talk about life: reproduction, metabolism and the ability to evolve'. (Boldt, Müller and Maio 2009, 47)

247) It is precisely as a whole that the organism then serves as a reference point for further research activities. It would appear that this ontological interpretation of a living organism as a whole can also be applied to a synthetically created organism. Although the initial conditions for its emergence are shaped by technological intervention, it subsequently behaves as a living biological system. Therefore, from the ontological viewpoint, there is no difference between this and a natural living organism, despite certain differences being observable at the ontogenesis or physiological level[4] (Gasser 2008, 144). Adopting this ontological position also allows us to avoid the potential ontological schism which would arise, Boldt, Müller and Maio argue, if we were to ascribe a different ontological status to artificial cells than that given to natural cells, for that would mean distinguishing "between two phenomenally and qualitatively similar cells". (Boldt, Müller and Maio 2009, 61) Since this also concerns artificial cells that go on to become living organisms, attempts to rename them, such as that by Nicole Karafyllis who labels artificial cells biofacts, do not fundamentally change the ontological interpretation. They just tighten up the terminology (Karafyllis 2003, 11–26). Indeed this ontological interpretation is in line with the existing research findings, based on which it is only possible to identify synthetic cells as an entirely new lifeform in a very narrow sense of the word, because the synthetic genome is still merely a copy of the natural genome sequence created during evolution. This means that their basic functions and properties correspond to those of a living organism (Bölker 2011, 32).

Determining the ontological status of synthetically created organisms is socially and culturally important because of the potential ethical consequences. We attribute value to living organisms from a particular point on the evolutionary scale, and this affects the way we treat them. Determining the ontological status of organisms, whose origin may have been technologically designed but whose subsequent development processes are similar to those occurring in natural organisms, will therefore decide whether we need to adjust our current ethical and value schemes in relation to nature. The ontological interpretation set out above does not require such a shift in boundaries when making ethical judgements.

[4] Where breeding or genetic modification is concerned, where changes are made to some of the properties of living organisms, the resulting organism is considered to be a *new version* of its natural predecessor (Deplazes-Zemp 2011, 100).

3. Anthropological interpretational images

In addition to the ontological questions there are also anthropological aspects associated with synthetic biology. If humans are capable not only of genetically altering existing lifeforms but also of creating the foundations for new life processes, the question arises as to whether this will change the existing image of humans and the way they see themselves.[5] Humans are self-interpreting beings who self-interpret from within a cultural-historical and scientific frame, based on relatively stable, but now changing forms of knowledge. However, the way humans understand themselves is often strong motivation for the search for further knowledge. Therefore, from the anthropological viewpoint there is reason to explore the kind of human image that has co-determined developments in modern bioscientific knowledge and whether this image is changing under the influence of current research in synthetic biology.

With the onset of modernity, the human ability to make, produce and manufacture gained primacy over other dispositions, and came to inform the anthropological image of *homo faber* (Arendt 2002, 377). The creative, active side of humans was largely manifested in the making of tools, and the tendency to imitate nature that had dominated ancient and medieval attitudes to the world was pushed into the background. With the tools they made, humans were able to expand knowledge and make nature more accessible so it could be put to effective use. Thus the new interpretation that was key to human self-understanding became the increasingly technical rationality that began to fundamentally shape scientific thinking and was behind many of the evolving scientific and technical projects (Müller 2009, 490). However, with the help of the converging technologies such a level of knowledge has been accumulated, as found in synthetic biology, that it goes far beyond that obtained using the old technological methods. The efforts to create new lifeforms, of a type not found thus far in nature, mean the evolutionary process has to be rationally controlled, unlike its previous form which merely required optimization and correction. Many writers, including Oliver Müller and Christoph Rehmann-Sutter, are therefore reflecting

[5] The expression 'human image' conveys the basic intuition that humans are formed within a broad historical, social and cultural context which enables them to self-interpret. For Oliver Müller one of the tasks in philosophical anthropology is to 'investigate the nature and boundaries of humans as a means of self-interpretation', precisely because human beings seek to self-understand (Müller 2009, 484).

on what the consequences of this new bioscientific knowledge might be for the anthropological image of humans and their self-interpretation. Just as human self-knowledge was in a certain way essential to the development of modern science, so modern science in the form of synthetic biology has the capacity to substantially influence human self-understanding.

Müller and Rehmann-Sutter differ in the arguments they present on how the human image is changing under the influence of research in synthetic biology. For Müller the driver of creativity and originality of humans as *homo faber*, and the main stimulus behind manufacturing, was the division between spirit and nature (Müller 2012, 226). However, synthetic biology has a creative impact on the natural process and hence disrupts this tension between the two. That means that while the traditional biotechnologies are still tied to the manufacturing model in which genetic manipulation is performed on nature in its current form, synthetic biology differs entirely. It is concerned with the more difficult task of creating the beginnings of entirely new artificial biological forms. It is for this reason that Müller suggests the manufacturing model is no longer adequate at this level. While manufacturing, or fabrication, was a means to an end, in the sense that it produced tools to exploit nature (Arendt 2002, 183), it seems the creativity of synthetic strategies is an end in itself, in the sense that it creates independently functioning synthetic systems. Müller therefore proposes that we should distinguish between the models of manufacturing and creation, and consequently this distinction is also linked to a gradual change in human self-understanding. The *homo faber* image that was conceived of in connection with manufacturing is being replaced by a new anthropological figure, *homo creator*,[6] a conception linked to *creatio a novo* (Müller 2012, 226).

Naturally this thesis is stimulating debate. This is being held at the level of re-assessing the anthropocentric position which has been further solidified by the strengthening of human competences in relation to the nature, as well as at the level of a more detailed examination of the relevance of the synthetic biology's results for the anthropological image. Christoph Rehmann-Sutter has undertaken an analysis of this relevancy, but instead of looking at the *homo creator* model he is more interested in *homo faber genomicus*, so that continuity can be maintained with the modernity project whilst avoiding theological objections (*playing God*) that do not get to

[6] Müller was inspired by the work of Günther Anders (*Die Antiquiertheit des Menschen*, München: Beck, 1980) and Hans Jonas (*Technik, Medizin und Ethik. Zur Praxis des Prinzips der Verantwortung*, Frankfurt am Main: Suhrkamp, 1987), who state that the spectrum of human ability has expanded to the extent that the *homo faber* model needs to be redefined. They base this assertion on their thinking about modern biotechnologies (Müller 2012, 223–224).

the heart of the problem (Rehmann-Sutter 2015, 30–31). Since philosophical anthropology does not explore the human being only in the sense of his difference from other living organisms, but also in the sense of his essence, the key question is whether we can regard the human capability of synthetically creating genome as new essence of the human, which would subsequently affect also his self-understanding. Rehmann-Sutter bases his argumentation on the difference between the delimitating definition of the human on the one hand and his essence on the other hand, i.e. on the difference between *quidditas* and *essentia* (Rehmann-Sutter 2015, 35). According to him it has not been sufficiently justified that the delimitating definition of the human vis-à-vis the realm of animals overlaps with what we regard as the essence of the human. While the delimitating process vis-à-vis other animal kinds is necessary for the definition of the human, it is not inevitable for the identification of his essence. Therefore he does not think that showing that no other animal is capable of synthetically creating a genome and proposing new lifeforms is sufficient to justify the notion of *homo faber genomicus*. This human peculiarity, specificity and uniqueness could come under *quidditas*, but that is not sufficient reason to equate this exclusive attribute with *essentia*. "I consider this path of self-interpretation of the human being through *quidditas* insufficient, because it prompts us to identify ourselves with those parts of ourselves, which set us apart from the rest of the nature (e.g. specifically qualified forms of self-consciousness, here: the biotechnological capability), while those parts that we have in common with other living organisms (e.g. sensation, consciousness, dependence on relationships) are defined as secondary". (Rehmann-Sutter 2015, 35–36) Rehmann-Sutter therefore sees no relevant reason for altering human self-interpretation simply because of synthetic biology research. Ultimately the ability to synthetically create a genome is restricted to a narrow circle of specialists and inaccessible to most people, and this undermines the idea that it changes the human image.[7]

[7] Rehmann-Sutter compares the human ability to synthetically create a genome with Plessner's Law of natural artificiality. It seems as if the new biotechnologies reflect Plessner's theory. If humans are not solidly biologically determined beings, then they have to shape themselves, and this could be interpreted as the need to shape and re-write their genetic make-up. However, Rehmann-Sutter does not think Plessner's Law concerns the ability to artificially interfere with nature and change the genetic code or synthesize a new one, but is about the ability to shape world culture via reflection. That means that *homo faber genomicus* cannot be seen as a continuation of Plessner's anthropological conception (Rehmann-Sutter 2015, 37–39).

On one hand, research in synthetic biology can be seen as the continuation, extension or even culmination of the technical rationality that is characteristic of the *homo faber* model and which is only now gaining an explicit form because of current research. According to this line of interpretation, it is not the shaping of a new human image that is key but rather the logical culmination of the modern anthropological model. On the other hand a range of opinions emphasize the difference between the existing methodological approaches used with classical biotechnologies on a prior lifeform and the technological strategies used in synthetic biology which are leading to the creation of new and hitherto non-existing biological systems. According to this interpretative stream the framework of human action in nature is expanding along with the framework of self-understanding. This is no longer simply about substituting for the biological inadequacies of human beings by manufacturing equipment that can be used to exploit nature effectively but about the ability to create and rationally design new (*de novo*) natural forms from scratch. It is this novelty in the natural sphere that is according to the second line of interpretation the motivation for extending or changing the anthropological image.

The fact that synthetic biology is still largely at the research stage and that the results can only be taken to indicate entirely new lifeforms in a limited sense (Bölker 2011, 32) favours the first line of interpretation more. If, however, we take a wider view and include anthropological thinking about extending the human competences in the sphere of human life and relating to other areas of contemporary bioscientific research, such as the transhumanist position on human enhancement,[8] then modern bioresearch cannot be overlooked in philosophical anthropology. There is no need to defend the notion of a powerful *homo creator* anthropological image, but clearly we cannot simply agree with the claim that new bioresearch is anthropologically irrelevant. Quite the opposite, greater attention should be paid to it at a time when we are starting to move away from the old order without there being a new one in place, for this is an era in which the old established boundaries are disappearing and the contours of the new ones are not yet clearly visible.

---

[8] Pharmacological brain altering substances and surgical modelling of the human body quickly became established in transhumanist enhancement. Attention has focused more recently on the possibility of genetically modifying information at both the somatic and germ levels, and on the potential to connect the human brain to equipment that can affect the actions of the nervous system. As a result, anthropological metaphors such as *posthuman* or *artificial life* abound.

Conclusion

Synthetic biology is a new research area linking the knowledge and technologies of various scientific and information disciplines. Its potential is being considered for the pharmaceutical industry in the manufacture of medicines and for environmental protection in the production of biological fuels or in the removal of harmful waste from the land (Bölker 2011, 40–41). As a new area of research it is naturally expanding both knowledge and the application opportunities on the one hand, whilst on the other giving rise to various legitimate questions. In this chapter, we have looked mainly at the ontological and anthropological questions associated with synthetic biology research. Using the work of G. Gasser we have attempted to show that despite the growing problems it is not possible to consider a synthetically created organism as an artefact. Although synthetic in origin, it later begins to display properties and evolution processes typical of a complex living organism, and so it can be ontologically interpreted as a whole similar to a natural living organism. This interpretation also allows us to avoid the potential ontological schism that would result if we were to differentiate between cells that have properties that are qualitatively the same in phenomenal terms. In terms of the anthropological line of thinking, two interpretative streams can be identified in relation to the new research in synthetic biology which reflect the influence new knowledge is having on the anthropological image of human beings. What is seen from one standpoint as new bioresearch simply extending the already established technical rationality, and therefore no reason to change the human self-interpretation, is for the other an approach that expands the framework of human competences such that it contributes to the formation of a new human image. The distinguishing criteria are created on the basis of new lifeforms. Although the current state of research in synthetic biology tends to favour the first idea more, we suggest that if we take other areas of bioscientific research into account one should not overlook the impact of the knowledge thus acquired on philosophical anthropology. This is despite the fact that the contours of the new identifying framework have yet to be fully drawn. In any case with the methods for designing new biological systems come high hopes that they will provide answers to fundamental questions about the functioning of life from the biological viewpoint.

Acknowledgement

This work was supported by Slovak Research and Development Agency contract No. APVV-0379-12.

Literature

Achatz, J. (2013) *Synthetische Biologie und „natürliche" Moral. Ein Beschreibungs- und Bewertungszugang zu den Erzeugnissen Synthetischer Biologie*, Freiburg, München: Karl Alber Verlag.

Arendt, H. (2002) *Vita activa oder Vom tätigen Leben*, München, Zürich: Piper Verlag.

Billerbeck, S. and Panke, S. (2012) Synthetische Biologie – Biotechnologie als eine Ingenieurwissenschaft, in Boldt, J., Müller, O. and Maio, G. (Eds): *Leben schaffen? Philosophische und ethische Reflexionen zur Synthetischen Biologie*, 19–40, Paderborn: Mentis Verlag.

Boldt, J. (2011) Natur 2.0? Zur Diskussion um die ethischen Aspekte der synthetischen Biologie, in Dabrock, P., Bölker, M., Braun, M. and Ried, J. (Eds): *Was ist Leben – im Zeitalter seiner technischen Machbarkeit? Beiträge zur Ethik der Synthetischen Biologie*, 309–326, Freiburg im Breisgau: Karl Alber Verlag.

Boldt, J. (2012) „Leben" in der Synthetischen Biologie: Zwischen gesetzesförmiger Erklärung und hermeneutischem Verstehen, in Boldt, J., Müller, O. and Maio, G. (Eds): *Leben schaffen? Philosophische und ethische Reflexionen zur Synthetischen Biologie*, 177–191, Paderborn: Mentis Verlag.

Boldt, J., Müller, O. and Maio, G. (2009) *Synthetische Biologie. Eine ethisch-philosophische Analyse*, Bern: Bundesamt für Bauten und Logistik.

Bölker, M. (2011) Revolution der Biologie? Ein Überblick über die Voraussetzungen, Ansätze und Ziele der Synthetischen Biologie, in Dabrock, P., Bölker, M., Braun, M. and Ried, J. (Eds): *Was ist Leben – im Zeitalter seiner technischen Machbarkeit? Beiträge zur Ethik der Synthetischen Biologie*, 27–41, Freiburg im Breisgau: Karl Alber Verlag.

Deplazes-Zemp, A. (2011) Leben als Werkzeugkasten. Die Auffassung von Leben in der Synthetischen Biologie, in Dabrock, P., Bölker, M., Braun, M. and Ried, J. (Eds): *Was ist Leben – im Zeitalter seiner technischen Machbarkeit? Beiträge zur Ethik der Synthetischen Biologie*, 95–115, Freiburg im Breisgau: Karl Alber Verlag.

Eichinger, T. (2011) Biodesign. Zu möglichen Abgrenzungskriterien der synthetischen Biologie von klassischer Gentechnik, in Dabrock, P., Bölker, M., Braun, M. and Ried, J. (Eds): *Was ist Leben – im Zeitalter seiner technischen Machbarkeit? Beiträge zur Ethik der Synthetischen Biologie*, 75–92, Freiburg im Breisgau: Karl Alber Verlag.

Gasser, G. (2008) Lebewesen und Artefakte. Ontologische Unterscheidungen, *Philosophisches Jahrbuch* 115 (1): 125–147.

Gibson, D. G. et al. (2010) Creation of a Bacterial Cell Controlled by a Chemically Synthesized Genome, *Science* 329 (5987): 52–56.

Heinemann, T. (2015) Leben als Konstrukt – Ethische Herausforderungen durch die Synthetische Biologie, in Rager, G. and Wegner, G. (Eds): *Synthetische Biologie – Leben als Konstrukt*, 229–266, Freiburg im Breisgau, München: Karl Alber Verlag.

Karafyllis, N. C. (2003) Das Wesen der Biofakte, in Karafyllis, N. C. (Ed): *Biofakte. Versuch über den Menschen zwischen Artefakt und Lebewesen*, 11–26, Paderborn: Mentis Verlag.

Mayr, E. (2002) Die Autonomie der Biologie, *Naturwissenschaftliche Rundschau* 55 (1): 23–29.

Müller, O. (2008) Der Mensch und seine Stellung zu seiner eigenen Natur. Zum Status anthropologischer Argumente in der bioethischen Debatte, in Maio, G., Clausen, J. and Müller, O. (Eds): *Mensch ohne Ma ? Reichweite und Grenzen anthropologischer Argumente in der biomedizinischen Ethik*, 15–57, Freiburg, München: Karl Alber Verlag.

Müller, O. (2009) Neurotechnologie und Menschenbild. Anmerkungen zu den anthropologischen Reflexionsfiguren Homo faber und Cyborg, in Müller, O., Clausen, J. and Maio, G. (Eds): *Das technisierte Gehirn. Neurotechnologien als Herausforderung für Ethik und Anthropologie*, 479–501, Paderborn: Mentis Verlag.

Müller, O. (2012) Vom Homo faber zum Homo creator? Synthetische Biologie und menschliches Selbstverständnis, in Boldt, J., Müller, O. and Maio, G. (Eds): *Leben schaffen? Philosophische und ethische Reflexionen zur Synthetischen Biologie*, 217–230, Paderborn: Mentis Verlag.

Rehmann-Sutter, C. (2015) „Remaking ourselves and our world" – Verändert die Synthetische Biologie die Rolle des Menschen?, in Baedke, J., Brandt, Ch. and Lessing, H.-U. (Eds): *Anthropologie 2.0? Neuere Ansätze einer philosophischen Anthropologie im Zeitalter der Biowissenschaften*, 25–44, Berlin: LIT Verlag.

Reth, M. (2012) Magie und Tragik der Synthetischen Biologie, in Boldt, J., Müller, O. and Maio, G. (Eds): *Leben schaffen? Philosophische und ethische Reflexionen zur Synthetischen Biologie*, 41–48, Paderborn: Mentis Verlag.

Sýkora, P. (2008) *Ontológia šera [Ontology in the Twilight]*, Trnava: Schola Philosophica.

Tomašovičová, J. (2018) Nové formy života? Filozofické reflexie syntetickej biológie [New Forms of Life? Philosophical Reflections on Synthetic Biology], *Filozofia* 73 (6): 437–448.

Venter, J. C. et al. (1995) The minimal gene complement of Mycoplasma genitalium, *Science* 270 (5235): 397–403.

Chapter 7

Germline genome editing and human nature

Peter Sýkora

Abstract: In the chapter I will explore the argument against radical human enhancement based on the natural law doctrine. Sitarčíková (2012) argues that it is necessary to protect human nature from huge (bio)technological interventions (human enhancement) since they will lead to a destruction of human nature. Due to it, humans will be deprived from the possibility to conduct right life and reach a final end of their existence, which is understanding of God. The argument can hardly be considered anything more than the application of Catholic moral doctrine of natural law. However, I will argue that Sitarcikova's argument (contrary to her own belief) makes sense even without God's existence premise. I will try to demonstrate that the doctrine of natural law and human nature with its final goal of human existence need not be religious and is in fact compatible with the natural science view of nature and humans.

Introduction[1]

The ethical consequences of the biotechnological manipulation of the human genome first began to be discussed in the late 1960s/early 1970s in relation to the emergence of new biotechnological tools that came to be associated with genetic engineering of recombinant DNA. Even in the early stages of debate, an important ethical distinction was made between somatic cell intervention and germline intervention (Anderson 1985, 1989). The genetic modification of somatic cells was viewed as an ethically uncontroversial approach that introduced the possibility of gene therapy for hereditary diseases. The reason for this was simple. Somatic gene therapy is performed within the medical paradigm - it concerns the treatment of a specific patient, albeit at the molecular level. It was seen as being in some way analogical to transplantation - not the transplantation of organs, tissue, or cells, but of genes. As originally conceived of, gene therapy simply involved the insertion of a foreign healthy gene into the cell of a patient to replace the function of the damaged gene.

However, unlike the consequences of interventions in somatic cell genes, those arising out of germline gene intervention, affecting the DNA of reproductive cells or early stage embryos, are passed on to subsequent

[1] This chapter is a substantial revision of the study Sýkora, P. (2014) Kritika teologicko-teleologickej koncepcie ľudskej prirodzenosti ako dôvodu odmietnutia transhumanizmu [Criticism of Theological-and-Teleological Concept of Human Nature as a Reason for Repudiating Transhumanism].

generations. Here it is not simply about treating a specific patient, as is the case in somatic gene therapy, but about treating potential patients who have yet to be born or even conceived. This in itself goes beyond the traditional medical paradigm. But in addition changes to *germline genes* are hereditary and can be passed on to future generations. While any undesirable effects of somatic gene therapy are restricted to the patient undergoing the treatment, those associated with germline gene interventions would become part of the hereditary make-up of future offspring.

To this day more than 2,000 clinical experiments involving somatic gene therapy have been conducted, and two somatic gene therapy–based medicines have been officially approved (Ginn et al. 2013). However, from 2003 to 2005 clinical trials were held on somatic gene therapy performed on boys with SCID-X1 (a severe combined immunodeficiency, known as 'bubble boy syndrome'). As a result of the treatment five of the 25 children developed leukaemia. Later analyses confirmed that the somatic cell gene therapy had led to the off-targeted insertions of the retroviral vector in the patient's DNA and the activating of proto-oncogenes due to it (Hacein-Bey-Abina et al. 2008). If this had occurred in germline gene therapy rather than somatic therapy, a new form of hereditary leukaemia would have been introduced into the human gene pool.

No wonder then that, since the debate began, any kind of germline gene intervention, whether for therapeutic purposes or to improve hereditary information, has been seen as totally unacceptable on the grounds that it represents a disproportionate health risk to future generations. Many countries around the world responded by explicitly banning interventions into human germline genes, either through national legislation or regulations (Araki and Ishii 2014), or via Article 13 of the European Convention on Human Rights and Biomedicine (The Oviedo Convention, 1997) which explicitly forbade any inheritable interventions in the human genome for the Council of Europe member states (like the Slovak Republic which signed and ratified it).

However, in the last five years the situation has changed dramatically with the emergence of gene editing technologies. These new biotechnological tools make it possible to edit the genetic information in DNA in much the same way as text is edited in word processing programs (hence the name of these technologies), through the targeted 'cut and paste' of DNA segments and spellchecking at the level of a single DNA base pair. Owing to its unprecedented precision, effectiveness, low cost, and technological simplicity, CRISPR/Cas9 is becoming the most popular gene editing platform. In 2015 Chinese scientists published the results of their ground-breaking, and as one might expect, highly controversial experiments, in which they successfully used CRISPR/Cas9 to edit the DNA of single-cell human embryos (zygotes) for the first time, thereby accomplishing the targeted modification of human germline genes (Liang et al. 2015).

The aim of this 'proof-of-principle' experiment was to demonstrate that CRISPR/Cas9, having been successfully applied in plants, animals, and human somatic cells, could also work in human embryonic cells, since it uses the natural DNA repair system in cells to function.

Genome editing technologies have of course also been used to create new genetically modified animals, or transgenic animals, especially in cases where traditional genetic engineering technologies are not sufficient, like in primates. Transgenic mice and rats with their simple nervous system cannot be used as animal models of neuropsychiatric disorders. Though it has proved possible to use directed gene editing to obtain transgenic cynomolgus monkeys (*Macaca fascicularis*) with precise mutations in selected genes (Niu et al. 2014). For the first time in history then, scientists have obtained, via gene editing platforms, the biotechnological tools to allow them to make targeted interventions in human DNA with previously unimaginable precision and technological ease, such that we can now realistically talk about the possibility of creating genetically modified people in the near future. Most scientists, as stem cell biologist, writer, and blogger Paul Knoepfler admits in the preface of his book *GMO Sapiens*, did not until recently take fears about genetically modified people seriously. This is because they were well aware of the huge technical roadblocks. However, gene editing technologies are fundamentally changing things because '[S]cience fiction is becoming reality in the biomedical world' (Knoepfler 2016).

Besides, it is probably only possible to rightfully talk about the potential emergence of a posthuman species, in the sense of a new biological species, what is the case of modified genetic information that is passed down to future generations, that is, the modification of germline genes. Cloaking ourselves in an exoskeleton in the way Iron Man the comic hero did, enabling us to fly, does not make us a member of a new biological species, for the simple and obvious reason that Iron Man's descendants will just be ordinary members of the Homo sapiens.

The entire discussion on human enhancement at the germline gene level is further complicated by the fact that scientists are far from agreed on *what* human nature is or *whether* such a thing as human nature in fact exists. Scholars from humanities and social sciences largely sit on one side with anti-essentialist attitudes in which human nature is considered to be a social and cultural construction.

On the other side we find the natural scientists whose prevailing view is that human nature is a set of fundamental characteristics and capabilities which humans have naturally and are genetically determined to greater or lesser degrees (also the subject of heated discussion). In other words, on this view human nature is encoded in human DNA. It is for this reason that biologists, for instance, suppose that in the minute differences between human and chimpanzee DNA, it is possible to find the answer to the question of 'what makes us human' (Pollard 2005).

From this it logically stems that tampering with germline genes, which have an important role to play in shaping this specifically human set of characteristics and capabilities, will ultimately lead to the end of original human nature by transforming it into a new posthuman 'nature'. Whether this change would be ethically acceptable is what lies at the heart of this disagreement.

In the Czech and Slovak intellectual sphere[2] the debate on the ethics of human enhancement has thus far been systematically covered in three monographs, two of which were published in the Czech Republic (M. Petrů 2005, Payne et al. 2015) and one in Slovakia (Sitarčíková 2012). In his extensive book M. Petrů argues in favour of human enhancement so long as the changes to the biological substrate lead to 'the human spirit developing in accordance with and on the basis of human values' (Petrů 2005, 246). He is of the opinion that caution is merited, but should not mean inaction. Just as the introduction of any technological innovation is a kind of social experiment, so human transformation will have to be introduced experimentally. But it will have to be performed under the condition of strict controls, as is in principle the case in liberal democracies (open societies), and be subjected to complex thinking (that takes account of the variability of reality and unexpected discoveries).

The second book is an edited monograph with contributions from ten authors (Payne et al. 2015) who consider human enhancement from various perspectives – philosophy, surgery, neurophysiology, genetics, cyborgs, doping, and the law. The authors' attitudes to human enhancement represent the entire ethical spectrum from liberal to conservative, but there is no reference to God or religious discourse. Most relevant to our own exploration of the relationship between human enhancement and human nature is A. Doležal's investigation of the law and its regulatory role. He

[2] Even after Czechoslovakia divided in 1993, Czech and Slovak intellectuals have continued to influence each other owing to their shared history and the proximity of the two languages.

approaches the issue from the perspective of positive law, within which the framework for the national regulation of new technologies, including human enhancement, will be set. Doležal does not consider human nature to be a social construct, but an objectively existing dynamic entity that exists despite our inability to define it, and one that we are nonetheless capable of working intuitively with. He defends the view that the 'gradual evolutionary' enhancement of human nature can be viewed as ethically acceptable, but not 'revolutionary transformation at the very core of human essence' (Payne et al. 2015, 147). He does not see germline interventions, including enhancement, as a problem in principle, so long as they do not involve revolutionary changes to germline genes: changes that would fundamentally transform human nature (Payne et al. 2015, 155–156).

While A. Doležal approaches the issue of human enhancement and human nature from the now dominant position of positive law, Z. Sitarčíková (2012), in her book *O šľachtení človeka - nanotechnológie, transhumanizmus a ľudská prirodzenosť* [*On human breeding: Nanotechnologies, transhumanism and human nature*], explores human enhancement from the standpoint of natural law theory, now generally considered to be dated. She takes her inspiration from the attempt by the well-known Czech Catholic thinker Stanislav Sousedík to justify the objectivity and universality of human rights by reviving the classical Thomist theory of natural law (Sousedík 2010). Sitarčíková applies this classical Thomist framework on human nature and natural law in her assessment of human enhancement. She concludes that radical human enhancement is ethically unacceptable because it would destroy human nature and thereby the meaning of human existence embedded within it.

My aim in this chapter is to show that Sitarčíková's argument on the need to protect human nature from enhancement is not, as she supposes, based on the premise of God's existence, but on the premise that human nature exists and that the final goal of human existence is stored within it, and that this is not necessarily dependent on the existence of God. For many these are one and the same: the existence of human nature with its predefined meaning of human life is unthinkable without reference to God the Creator. On the other hand, for majority of scholars in humanities and social sciences, human nature does not exist. However, if the existence of human nature is accepted, which is more the view of natural scientists, then it definitely does not contain a final goal or the meaning of human existence hidden within it, since for modern science there is no pre-existing final goal of anything in nature. Modern natural science, established in the sixteenth to seventeenth centuries, rejects the teleological view of nature that explains natural events by reference to Aristotle's *causa finalis*.

Despite this common view I will argue that when discussing human enhancement one should also consider the modern, 'updated' version of the naturalized, post-Darwinian conception of human nature along with the 'updated' view of the purpose (*telos*) of the existence of living organisms, including human existence.

Protecting human nature argument

In the expert debates that have now been going on with varying degrees of intensity for more than four decades, the impact of the potential modification of human germlines in terms of safety and the religious, ethical, and social consequences had already been analysed in detail before genome editing techniques were discovered.[3] In principle there are two opposing camps. On one side stand those who welcome the possibility of the targeted modification of human genetic nature. They hold that human nature, formed during evolution through blind natural forces, is far from perfect (e.g. Harris 2007, Buchanan 2011, Mehlman 2012, Bostrom and Sandberg 2009). They see no reason to consider human DNA as a sacred and taboo entity that cannot be touched. Harris (2007) says that it would have been equally absurd to try and prevent Australopithecus from continuing to evolve into Homo sapiens in the name of preserving Australopithecus nature. On the contrary, genetic human enhancement can be seen as a further stage in human evolution, in which the role of the ineffective, slow, and blind process of natural evolution is replaced with a purposeful, effective, rapid redesigning of human genome.

On the other side are those who reject germline gene intervention in humans. They have several reasons for doing so. Until recently the strongest argument was the prohibitively high risks associated with the imprecision of traditional genetic engineering methods. This argument will lose strength as gene editing becomes safer.

It is worth noting here that not everyone supposes that genetic methods of human enhancement are ethically different from other biological

[3] For example, Friedmann and Robin 1972, Anderson 1989, Resnick et al. 1999, Campbell and Stock 2000, Rasko et al. 2006, Smith et al. 2012.

and non-biological forms of enhancement (Buchanan 2011). Nonetheless in the context of creating genetically modified organisms at least, there is a considerable difference between enhancing human germline genes and all other forms of human enhancement. Not to mention that when viewed historically, modification of the human germline has to be seen within the context of the eugenic practices of the first half of the twentieth century. Unlike genetic enhancement, chemical and cyborg methods of enhancement have nothing to do with eugenics.

One of the most important and most discussed objections to human germline interventions is the need to protect human nature as part of our common natural heritage. Human genetic nature has to be seen as a natural complex system. We do not have the requisite knowledge to be able to change this complex system responsibly and without risk, however justified our intentions are. It is a biological fact that the human genome acquired its current form as a complex system as a result of long years of biological evolution during which its genes began to mutually operate in synchronization such that it forms a balanced whole. Any, even well-intentioned, interventions into such a system, albeit small ones, may disrupt its balance, causing the entire complex system to break down. According to a well-known report by the US President's Council on Bioethics (Kaas 2003) we will have to learn from the unfortunate environmental consequences of people's well-intentioned, but insufficiently knowledgeable, attempts to intervene in ecosystems, which are another kind of fragile natural complex system. Incompetent interventions into complex systems almost always lead not to improvement, but to destruction. This is even recognized by the most enthusiastic defenders of enhancing and altering human nature, who have great respect for the 'Wisdom of Mother Nature' embedded in the human genome (Bostrom and Sandberg, 2009).

Another argument favouring the protection of human nature points out that the concept of universal human rights relies upon the idea there is a common universal human nature. Destroying human nature would not simply threaten human rights, but undermine democratic political institutions which are grounded on them (Fukuyama 2002). Several objectors to human germline gene intervention base their arguments on the unfortunate historical experiences of eugenics in the twentieth century. Allowing the genetic enhancement of people would enable the creation of a human subpopulation ('race') or even a new human biological species that would be superior thanks to the biological dispositions for longevity, better health, amazing cognitive abilities, and so forth, which would mean that existing non-enhanced humans would be at a disadvantage and would therefore become enslaved and end up being eliminated (Ramsey 1970, Annas 2002).

By contrast supporters of enhancement (transhumanists) consider human inequality arising from enhancement to be a social problem, rather than an inherently technological one. They argue that one can assume that genetic enhancement will rapidly become accessible to all, as has been the case with mobile phones, and that everyone will benefit from its advantages (Harris 2007). Others object, saying that this is naïve, since it ignores negative historical experiences, and that so long as there is a tool that will potentially allow people to control others, then that tool is highly likely to be abused (Sparrow 2014).

The religious view occupies a category of its own in this debate on protecting human nature against technological intervention. It centres around the 'playing God' argument which holds that humans were created by God, and that it is therefore inappropriate to perfect God's creation. People do not have the requisite knowledge and never will. Only all-powerful God has that knowledge. It is a biblical myth stretching from the forbidden fruit on the tree of knowledge to human pride (hubris), reinforced through God's command. In this respect it is worth noting that some modern theologians question this argument by pointing to the assumption on which it is based: that God considers human nature to be perfect, to be his final creation. Theologically, Peterson (2010, 87) argues this 'neglects the effects of sin or the possibility that the first humans were the starting point, not the grand finale of God's intent'.

With the *emerging genome editing technologies* we find ourselves in a new situation. For the first time it is not simply a theoretical possibility. This can be seen in the exceptionally quick reaction of the international academic community to the attempt by Chinese scientists to edit the genes of human embryos. Before the research was published, a modest group of prominent American scientists and bioethicists met in Napa, California, to discuss the newly developed situation. At the meeting they agreed on a statement (later published in *Science* by Baltimore et al. 2015), in which they warned against rushing into the use of human germline gene editing in clinical practice, but they did not rule out basic research in the field.

Another group of American scientists produced a far more radical statement which was published in *Nature*. It called for a moratorium on any kind of attempt at germline gene editing in humans, not just in clinical research, but in basic research too (Lanphier et al. 2015). However, both groups explicitly supported and stressed the enormous potential of gene editing technologies for use in *somatic cell gene therapy*.

Throughout 2015 various scientific, professional and *policy forming* organizations across the world made statements on *genome editing in humans*. The discussions culminated in the International Summit on Human Gene Editing in December 1–3, in Washington, DC, organized by the National Academy of Sciences and the National Academy of Medicine's Human Gene-Editing Initiative and co-hosted with the Chinese Academy of Sciences and the UK's Royal Society. An international expert group was set up at the summit to assess the scientific, ethical, and governance issues associated with human genome editing. Fourteen months later the commission presented its 261-page report on *Human Genome Editing: Science, Ethics, and Governance* (NASEM 2017), which most surprisingly permitted germline gene intervention in humans for therapeutic reasons so long as they were subjected to extensive research aimed at meeting the existing risk/benefit standards for clinical trials. However, the commission was uncompromising in its rejection of genome editing for enhancement purposes. The media labelled this a red-to-yellow 'traffic light' change in biopolicy (Kaiser 2017).

Natural law argument against radical human enhancement

We will now consider Z. Sitarčíková's argument against intervening in human nature because it could destroy the meaning of human life.

The very title of Sitarčíková's book *O šľachtení človeka – nanotechnológie, transhumanizmus a ľudská prirodzenosť* [*On human breeding: nanotechnologies, transhumanism and human nature*] indicates her negative view of transhumanist attempts at enhancing the human species through the use of modern technologies, since the term *šľachtenie človeka* [human breeding] is associated with the negative connotations of eugenics. The aim of her book, according to the author, is to justify why we should '(continue) prioritizing *zušľachťovanie* over *šľachtenie*' (p. 14, italics in original).

The Slovak terms "zušľachťovanie" and "šľachtenie" have the same word root of "šlachta" (nobility). The word "šlachtenie" is equivalent to the English term "breeding" and it refers to the genetic 'bloodline' of the aristocracy, in much the same way as genetic lines or varieties of animals or plants are bred; while "zušľachťovanie" means ennobling – cultivation, upbringing, raising a person to have good manners, etc. Sitarčíková's whole argument turns on a contrast between human 'breeding' (šlachtenie), albeit in the broader sense of the radical technological enhancement of humans, as opposed to ennobling (zušľachťovanie). She thinks the former is unacceptable, whereas the latter is acceptable to the humanist tradition, and also, in fact, a moral imperative.

Sitarčíková uses the term *šľachtenie* to refer to various forms of human enhancement, not just genetic or biomedical enhancement, but also the cyborgization of the human body or nanotechnology-based interventions or with new synthetic chemical substances. The important point here is the extent to which the intervention changes human nature. If it changes it fundamentally, as does for example radical enhancement – the goal of transhumanists, then this is *šlachtenie*, ethnically undesirable human breeding: the creation of a new posthumanist species. Genetic interventions, unlike other interventions such as nanotechnological ones, play a crucial role here because they do not just radically change human nature at the individual level but change the human biological species as a whole (Sitarčíková 2012, 45–46). Sitarčíková is not completely against all technological interventions in the human body. They are acceptable insofar as they do not change human nature, but simply repair it if damaged, and insofar as the interventions are minor ones performed within the limits of the human species.

Sitarčíková believes that radical technological interventions aimed at human enhancement destroy the metaphysical union between the spiritual and bodily components that make up human nature and therefore deprive humans of the meaning of their existence, which is above all about knowing God and loving one's nearest and dearest. Given what she says, her argument requires one to accept the premise of God's existence. However, she does not consider her argument to be religious or theological, but philosophical. In truth she does not refer to religious faith, the Bible, or religious authority in her argument. Indeed her premise on the existence of God, which she considers essential, is presented as a philosophical one, which means it does not rely on religion but on modern, logical, and metaphysical proof of God's existence. She attempts to find purely rational, or empirical, justification for all her premises, including those about the existence of God and about the metaphysical character of human nature, not religious or theological justification. She refers to biology or to philosophical analyses of human nature like those of H. Arendt or V. Frankel's psychological analysis of suffering. Apart from one, albeit substantial, exception: her definition of human nature. For this she seeks the assistance of Pope John Paul II's encyclical *Veritatis Splendor* (see below).

The conceptual frame of Sitarčíková's argument is formed out of the classical Thomist theory of natural rights and human nature. According to Czech philosopher S. Sousedík, whom Sitarčíková relies upon exclusively in relation to this issue, the meaning of human life is to adhere to natural law, which leads us to know God and love for other people, and from this it stems that:

> 'If, however, we want to know God, we have to get close to him, and getting close to him means respecting his will, which is inscribed in human nature through natural law (Sousedík 2010, 77–78).'

The existence of universal human nature is therefore crucial to the universal validity of natural law, because it is only thanks to common human nature that an objective natural law that is valid for all people can exist. Sousedík's thesis is that in today's situation it is possible to justify the binding respect for human rights only by reinstating the concept of natural law and universal human nature, without which universal natural rights are unthinkable (Sousedík 2010, 9–10). This means that all natural entities (animals, plants, minerals), including humans, have a nature/essence specific to that species, created through natural propensities or *inclinations*. With the exception of humans, everything is controlled through these natural propensities or inclinations. Since humans have their own free will they can, but needn't, behave in accordance with their natural inclinations. Behaving in accordance with natural inclinations is the substance of natural law. According to Sousedík the greatest natural inclination 'is to know God to the greatest degree possible (and love stems from that)' (Sousedík 2010, 78). Achieving this greatest inclination is therefore the goal, the meaning, of human life.

Sitarčíková's argument goes like this:

P1: God, the creator of all entities, exists.
P2a: God gives each entity created its nature and he also gives humans their human nature.
P2b: There exists a universal human nature/essence that is common to all people because without this concept discussions on posthumanism would make no sense.
P3: A number of natural human inclinations exist in human nature and it is through these that humans fulfil their final (ultimate) goal and the meaning of their existence.
P4: The most important human inclination is to know God.

P5: Radical interventions in human nature change human nature, which is the equivalent of destroying it.
P6: The disappearance of human nature means the loss of natural inclinations, including the inclination to know God, which means that humans lose their ultimate goal and meaning of their existence.
P7: Human life in which existence has no meaning is ethically unacceptable.
C: Radical interventions into human nature are ethically unacceptable because they lead to the destruction of human nature and thereby the meaning of human existence is lost as well.

Critical evaluation of Sitarčíková's argument based on natural law and human nature

First of all we should note that Sitarčíková considers the premise relating to God to be central to her argument, since she states: 'Understandably we are conscious of the fact that this argument is only acceptable if we accept the existence of God as its premise, [...]'. (Sitarčíková 2012, 171 - Footnote. 483). But that would mean the argument is only valid for those who believe in monotheistic religions. Sitarčíková, however, sees it differently. She adopts the conception of God that Sousedík uses in his attempt to justify the binding nature of universal human rights. In his view (and that of Sitarčíková), God is not the object of faith but is a rationally known entity (Sousedík 2010, 31). Sousedík admits that he is a 'Catholic Christian and ascribes great value to his faith', but says he wants to deliberately distance himself from his faith and think on rational grounds only (Sousedík 2010, 73). He suggests that two modern pieces of evidence for the existence of God (from K. Goedel and R. Swinburn) allow us to accept, in a purely philosophical manner, that God really exists in the sense he is perceived to by the great monotheistic religions such as Judaism, Christianity, and Islam (Sousedík 2010, 74). The argument that God exists is therefore valid for all rationally thinking people and not only for the believers of traditional monotheistic religions.

The basic question relating to this argument on protecting human nature against technological intervention is whether there is such a thing as human nature. And if so, whether it contains the natural inclinations that lead humans to fulfil the meaning of their existence. As we have already mentioned, Sitarčíková's reliance on the papal encyclical when defining human nature undermines her claim to be pursuing a non-religious argument. Subscription to the official Roman Catholic moral doctrine, reliant upon the natural law conception of God and of God as the ultimate goal of human existence, is presented as a fact. Yet she herself provides further justification for the existence of human nature (premise P2b). In this premise Sitarčíková sees proof of the existence of human nature coming from the meaningfulness of the debate surrounding it. If we talk of transforming human nature, be it from the supporting or opposing side, then we can only suppose that 'there is someone who knows what human nature is, what transforming it means and whether it is at all possible' (Sitarčíková 2012, 152). This semantic reason for the existence of human nature would appear to have seemed weaker to her than the authority of the papal office.

Sitarčíková's view of the nature of entities is entirely Platonic: 'Everything has its own nature–essence–without which it would not be what it is' (Sitarčíková 2012, 155). Just as all triangles share one and the same essence - 'they have three angles' - and it is this which makes them what they are, that is, triangles. A triangle without three angles cannot be called a triangle. Similarly, all people have the same human nature/essence, which makes them people. There are a "certain number of characteristics common to all people without distinction, based on which they can be labelled as 'human'" (Sitarčíková 2012, 155). Nature does not change, because the metaphysical principle of unity between body and soul is fixed, which Sitarčíková explains thus: 'To say that human nature thus conceived of can change is like saying that a square whose angles have been altered changes into a circle' (Sitarčíková 2012, 165–166). She seems to be saying that a tangible square can change into another geometric shape through deformation, but these changes in no way affect the metaphysical essence of the triangle.

The metaphysical essence of a human is, according to Pope John Paul II's Encyclical *Veritatis Splendor*, paragraph 50, 'the person himself in the unity of soul and body, in the unity of his spiritual and biological inclinations and of all the other specific characteristics necessary for the pursuit of his end' (Sitarčíková 2012, 165).

Sitarčíková understands indivisibility to mean that human nature cannot be reduced to its cultural or spiritual components, nor to its biological, genetic, or material elements. In this regard she is critical of O. Wilson's sociobiological approach to human nature, which she thinks reduces the cultural and social dimensions of humans to mere biology. Sitarčíková considers the material basis of heredity to be so flexible (she is thinking of epigenetic heredity here) that it is not possible for it to be human nature.

She bases her claim that human nature cannot be reduced to a purely spiritual or cultural element on the fact that we know that the human ability to learn a human language comes from the human genome and is not cultural. But fundamental to her view of human nature is that it is a metaphysical entity:

> 'We do not therefore understand human nature to be something measurable or specific, like DNA for instance, but as a metaphysically conceived principle of the unity of body and soul (Sitarčíková 2012, 165).'

Sitarčíková provides an example of the destruction of human nature in which human consciousness is uploaded onto a computer, and all the human psychological (spiritual) characteristics are stored (on the computer), but the biological and spiritual unity is destroyed in the process and thus, she believes, the metaphysical unity of the biological and spiritual as well. Another example in which human nature is destroyed is the radical enhancement of human abilities such as acquiring the ability to see in the dark or live under water. Since these go beyond the limits of the world of human biology, they destroy human nature (Sitarčíková 2012, 168–169). By contrast more moderate forms of what Sitarčíková calls 'disembodied existence', such as brain implants to enhance memory or concentration, do not destroy human nature since they do not go beyond the boundaries of the 'biological human world'.

But Sitarčíková's view of human nature lacks coherence. On the one hand, she understands human nature to mean the metaphysical unity of body and spirit in humans, which she compares ontologically to the Platonic Form of the triangle or square, and on the other she talks about its destruction. However, by definition the Platonic Forms cannot be destroyed! Put differently, how can a technological tool from the changeable 'world of shadows' destroy Platonic metaphysical human nature?

Sitarčíková claims that her argument is a philosophical one because it assumes God's existence can be rationally explained, but in fact her argument applies official Christian moral doctrine to technological human enhancement. Reasons found in empirical sciences, such as biology, are deliberately selected and moreover are then mistakenly and incoherently interpreted, as I have shown elsewhere (Sýkora 2014). For instance, she justifies her claim that human nature cannot be stored in DNA because genetic inheritance is too variable by referring to the phenomenon of epigenetic inheritance. Yet she ignores the relatively high degree of stability shown by biological species (so stable in fact that people were not able to accept evolutionary change) that is achieved because of the even greater stability displayed by genes.

Human nature, telos, natural law, and ethics – all naturalized

The main objection human scientists make is that the information that makes humans human cannot be stored in genes because it is found in human spirituality rather than in biology. The latest research, however, shows that the relationship between the spiritual and biological sides of being human is far closer than human and social scientists are generally willing to accept. Pinker's book *The Blank Slate* maps out in detail this shift from the humanist and social paradigm of the *tabula rasa* to the far more complex idea that inner biology and the genetic components of human nature combine with elements of the external environment (Pinker 2002).

For example, extensive systematic research by psychologists, in which they investigated, using standard tests, the cognitive, emotional, and personal characteristics of monozygotic twins who had been separated at birth and brought up in different families, revealed a surprisingly high proportion of genetic components in the test results (Plomin et al. 1997).

It is important to stress here that the genetic basis of human nature only determines a specific general framework of human behaviour, not the specific form it takes. That emerges through interaction with the environment. However, the genetic basis means we can refer to inclinations, dispositions, and *capabilities*. These are then shaped and moulded and realized under the influence of the social and cultural environment. A paradigmatic example of human nature thus conceived is human language. There exists an innate human ability to acquire language, but it is the environment, not genes, that determines which language that will be.

There has long been speculation that natural law could have natural rather than religious origins. Morality, until recently considered an exclusively cultural phenomenon, can have a partly neurobiological basis. Here one might mention the ethical brain (Gazaniga 2005), the fact that love for those dear to us may be an innate inclination to altruistic behaviour (Katz 2000, Tomasello 2016) that comes not from God but from Darwinian natural selection, and that natural law may be a product of evolution (Arnhart 1998). Arnhart argues extensively that 'the moral sense is natural, it does not *require* religious belief, although religious belief can *reinforce* the moral sense' (Arnhart 1998, 249; his emphasis).

This would mean that the universality of human nature and certain moral principles were the result of a genetically determined neurobiological set-up of the brain common to all people. The variability of different moral systems across time and space - an argument frequently used by human scientists against universal natural law - could then be explained as the result of the same inner and genetically conditioned moral equation, but dependent upon various external, social, historical, and cultural input parameters that generate various outcomes and various specific moralities (Hauser 2006).

If the concept of natural law is to be fully naturalized, then in addition to explaining the evolutionary origins of human inclinations to moral behaviour, it has to explain human existence as the ultimate goal. Since the seventeenth century the final goal has been considered a synonym for dated, unscientific explanations for phenomena in nature. However, just as Darwinism can provide a new explanatory framework for understanding the stark contrast between purposefulness in living nature and blind causal natural processes, so too can it explain the existence of purposefulness in living nature. As Arnhart quipped (2011) '[E]ven if evolution by natural selection is not purposeful, it produces organic beings that are purposeful. Plants and animals grow to maturity, and once grown, they act for ends set by the functional nature of each species' (Arnhart 2011, 44).

One of the pioneers who began 'updating' purposeful causes in biology was the well-known zoologist and philosophical biologist Ernst Mayr working in the mid-1970s. In order to banish the awkward misunderstandings and to distinguish new conceptions of teleology from traditional, idealistic, or psychological content, he decided on a new term - teleonomy. Mayr argues that there are purposeful, teleonomic processes and activities going on at different levels in living nature. These goal-directed processes, activities, and behaviours exist thanks to a genetic programme created through biological evolution (Mayr 2009).

Mayr compared the genetic programme controlling the ontogenesis of the organism to Aristotle's *causa finalis*. The aim of evidently purposeful processes such as embryogenesis and the subsequent development of the individual is present right from the start. The *telos* of each embryogenesis is stored in the DNA of a fertilized egg. To various degrees the behaviour of an organism is thus predetermined. We now know that the species-specific morphology, anatomy, physiology, and behaviour of organisms is the result of the blind natural forces of Darwin's evolutionary process.

On this view then we can quite legitimately now ask what kind of *telos* was formed during the evolution of our biological species. One answer is provided by Aristotle in *The Nicomachean Ethics* and in *The Eudemian Ethics*, and that is the function argument. According to Aristotle, humans have a specific function (*to ergon tou anthropou*), which has to be fulfilled, realized, in the most excellent (excellence = virtue) manner because it will bring them happiness (*eudaimonia*) (Johnson 2005, 211–222). So, what is this specific human function? Aristotle thought it was using reason, in the sense that practical reason leads people to live a full life in a community of people, in a *polis*. So above all it is about using the theoretical reason which enables us to understand reality in its essence. As Aristotle famously said at the beginning of his *Metaphysics* 'all men by nature desire to know' (Met 1.1.), not just any kind of knowledge, but theoretical knowledge. In other words people are naturally inclined to discover the essence of the world. This innate, and therefore genetically determined, inclination to theoretically comprehend the world, which is manifested in its purest form in mathematics or metaphysics, is, Aristotle believes, the truly ultimate goal (*telos*) of human existence. If this cognitive inclination to understand the abstract essence of the world, identified as God in the religious tradition, is innate, then seeking out God is an innate inclination ('the God gene').

In this whole discussion, it is important to distinguish between the Platonic cosmic teleology rejected by modern science and Aristotle's immanent theology of living organisms, which also concerns the human biological species. At the same time it must be stressed that innate human inclination, genetic predisposition, comes nowhere near as close to determining human life in the rigid way it does animal life. Humans typically possess an unprecedented flexibility in fulfilling their biological potential or capacities. Empirical researchers are still faced with the enormous challenge of detailing the relationship between the very open biological frames, potentialities, capacities, and inclinations of human nature on the one hand and the flexible, variability of their actual realization under the influence of the cultural and social environment on the other.

Conclusion

The argument set out by the Slovak author Z. Sitarčíková against attempts at radical human enhancement hinge factually on the official

Catholic doctrine of natural law and the final goal of human existence, which is to know God. It is basically a religious argument, despite the author's declarations that it is philosophical in character, since it stems from the religious moral doctrine of natural law and human nature. To portray this argument as a philosophical one is therefore misleading. It is not a theological argument either because it is not framed within the theological discourse on human enhancement (as is for instance the work of Peterson 2010).

In addition to analysing Sitarčíková's argument, which can hardly be considered anything more than the application of Catholic moral doctrine of natural law, I have attempted to demonstrate that the doctrine of natural law and human nature with its final goal of human existence need not be religious and is in fact compatible with the natural science view of nature and humans.

In the naturalized conception of human nature, natural law, and (biological) purposefulness, genetic information is passed down from generation to generation through germline genes, and substantially determines the framework within which specific human dispositions and capacities, intuitively seen as human nature, are realized under the influence of the environment. It logically ensues from this that interventions into human germline genes may alter human nature. For decades, interventions into human *germline genes* were simply not an issue, largely because of the enormous potential health risks that could affect future generations. That all changed in 2015 when a group of Chinese scientists announced they had successfully modified human germline genes using CRISPR/CAS9 gene editing. It is true that thus far this technology has not met the *safety* standards applicable to clinical use (the concern mainly being the undesirable generation of *off-target effects*), but we are seeing unprecedentedly rapid progress in terms of effectiveness and precision of this technology. Experts expect a level of precision that would make clinical trials on genome editing in humans acceptable to be achieved soon.

In ethics discussions, the distinction between heritable genetic enhancement and other forms of enhancement is not frequently made because ethical judgements concentrate on *human attributes and abilities*. This may well also be related to the dominant paradigm in the humanities and social sciences that holds that human nature does not exist and that genes are not important for the determination of typical human attributes and abilities. Ethics discussions tend to deal with the scope of enhancement rather than the manner in which it is achieved. A number of authors consider radical enhancement to be unethical since it involves improving human attributes and abilities to levels that greatly exceed what is currently possible for human beings.

If, for the sake of argument, we accept the opinion that the final goal/ meaning of human existence, which is the ability to think theoretically ('metaphysically'), has a genetic basis, then the fear that germline gene intervention may disrupt or destroy this ability is justified. In other words, the fear that intervening in human germline genes may deprive humans of the meaning of life exists independently from the acceptance of God or of cosmic teleology concepts.

Acknowledgement

This work was supported by Slovak Research and Development Agency contract No. APVV-0379-12.

Literature

Agar, N. (2010) *Humanity's End: Why We Should Reject Radical Enhancement*, Cambridge: MIT Press.

Anderson, W. F. (1985) Human Gene Therapy: Scientific and Ethical Considerations, *Journal of Medicine and Philosophy* 10, 275–291.

Anderson, W. F. (1989) Human Gene Therapy: Why Draw a Line? *Journal of Medicine and Philosophy* 14, 681–693.

Annas, G. J., Andrews, L. B. and Isasi, R. M. (2002) Protecting the Endangered Human: Toward an International Treaty Prohibiting Cloning and Inheritable Alterations, *American Journal of Law and Medicine* 28 (2/3), 151–178.

Araki, M. and Ishii T. (2014) International Regulatory Landscape and Integration of Corrective Genome Editing into in vitro Fertilization, *Reproductive Biology and Endocrinology* 12, 108–120.

Arnhart, L. (1998) *Darwinian Natural Right: The Biological Ethics of Human Nature*, Albany: State University of New York Press.

Baltimore, D., Berg, P., Borchan, M., et al. (2015) A Prudent Path Forward for Genomic Engineering and Germline Gene Modification, *Science* 248 (6230), 36–38.

Bostrom, N. and Sandberg, A. (2009) The Wisdom of Nature: An Evolutionary Heuristic for Human Enhancement, in Savulescu, J. and Bostrom, N. (Eds) *Human Enhancement*, Oxford: Oxford University Press, 375–416.

Buchanan, A. (2011) *Beyond Humanity?: The Ethics of Biomedical Enhancement*, Oxford: Oxford University Press.

Campbell, J. and Stock, G. (2000) A Vision for Practical Human Germline Engineering, in Stock, G. and Campbell, J. (Eds) *Engineering the Human Genome: An Exploration of the Science and Ethics of Altering the Genes We Pass to Our Children*, Oxford: Oxford University Press, 9–16.

Friedman, T. and Robin, R. (1972) Gene Therapy for Human genetic Disease? *Science* 175 (4025), 949–955.

Fukuyama, F. (2002) *Our Posthuman Future: Consequences of the Biotechnological Revolution*, New York: Farrar, Straus and Giroux.

Gazzaniga, M. (2005) *The Ethical Brain: The Science of Our Moral Dilemmas*, New York: HarperCollins Publishers.

Ginn, S. L., Alexander, I. E., Edelstein, M. L., et al. (2013) Gene Therapy Clinical Trials Worldwide to 2012 – An Update, *The Journal of Gene Medicine* 15, 65–77.

Hacein-Bey-Abina, S., Garrigue, A., Wang, G. P., et al. (2008) Insertional Oncogenesis in 4 Patients After Retrovirus-Mediated Gene Therapy of SCID-X1, *Journal of Clinical Investigation* 118 (9), 3132–3142.

Harris, J. (2007) *Enhancing Evolution: The Ethical Case for Making Better People*, Princeton: Princeton University Press.

Hauser, M. (2006) *Moral Minds: How Nature Designed Our Universal Sense of Right and Wrong*, New York: HarperCollins Publishers.

Johnson, M. R. (2005) *Aristotle on Teleology*, Oxford: Clarendon Press.

John Paul II (1993) *Encyclical Letter Veritatis Splendor*, Vatican City: Libreria Editrice Vaticana.

Kaas, L., Blackburn, E., Dresser, R. S., et al. (2003) *Beyond Therapy: Biotechnology and the Pursuit of Happiness*, Washington DC: President's Council on Bioethics.

Kaiser, J. (2017) U.S. panel gives yellow light to human embryo editing. *Science Magazine News* (Feb.14, 2017), available online: http://www.sciencemag.org/news/2017/02/us-panel-gives-yellow-light-human-embryo-editing. (Access: 14.06.2017)

Katz, L. D. (Ed) (2000) *Evolutionary Origins of Morality: Cross-Disciplinary Perspectives*, Bowling Green: Imprint Academic.

Knoepfler, P. (2015) *GMO Sapiens: The Life-Changing Science of Designer Babies*, Singapore: World Scientific Publishing Company.

Lanphier, E., Urnov, F., Haecker, S. E., et al. (2015) Don't Edit the Human Germ Line, *Nature* 519, 410–411.

Liang, P., Xu, Y., Zgang, X., et al. (2015) CRISPR/Cas9-Mediated Gene Editing in Human Triponuclear Zygotes, *Protein Cell* 6 (5), 363–372.

Mayr, E. (2004) *What Makes Biology Unique?: Considerations on the Autonomy of a Scientific Discipline*, Cambridge: Cambridge University Press.

Mehlman, M. J. (2012) *Transhumanist Dreams and Dystopian Nightmares: The Promise and Peril of Genetic Engineering*, Baltimore: The John Hopkins University Press.

National Academies of Sciences, Engineering, and Medicine (NASEM 2017) *Human*

Genome Editing: Science, Ethics, and Governance, Washington DC: The National Academies Press.

Niu, Y., Shen, B., Cui, Y., et al. (2014) Generation of Gene-Modified Cynomolgus Monkey via Cas9/RNA-Mediated Gene Targeting in One-Cell Embryos, *Cell* 156, 836–843.

Payne, J., Černý, D., Doležal, A., et al. (2015) *Dobrý, nebo lepší život?: Human Enhancement*, Praha: Ústav státu a práva AVČR, v.v.i.

Peterson, J.C. (2010) *Changing Human Nature. Ecology, Ethics, Genes, and God*, Grand Rapids, Michigan: Wm.B. Eerdmans Publishing Co.

Petrů, M. (2005) *Možnosti transgrese: Je třeba vylepšovat člověka?*, Praha: Triton.

Pinker, S. (2002) *The Blank Slate*, New York: Viking.

Plomin, R., DeFries, J. C., McClearn, G. E. and Rutter, M. (Eds.) (1997) *Behavioral Genetics* (3rd edition), New York: W.H. Freeman and Company.

Pollard, K. S. (2009) What Makes Us Human? *Scientific American* 300 (5), 44–49.

Ramsey, P. (1970) *Fabricated Man: The Ethics of Genetic Control*, Yale: Yale University Press.

Rasko, J. E., O´Sullivan, G. M. and Ankeny, R. A. (Eds) (2006) *The Ethics of Inheritable Genetic Modification: A Dividing Line?*, Cambridge: Cambridge University Press.

Resnik, D. B., Steinkraus H. B. and Langer P. J. (1999) *Human Germline Gene Therapy: Scientific, Moral and Political Issues*, Austin: R.G. Landes Company.

Sitarčíková, Z. (2012) *O šľachtení človeka: Nanotechnológie, transhumanizmus a ľudská prirodzenosť*, Trnava: Typi Universitatis Tyrnaviensis.

Smith, K. R., Chan, S. and Harris, J. (2012) Human Germline Genetic Modifications: Scientific and Bioethical Perspective, *Archives of Medical Research* 43, 491–513.

Sousedík, S. (2010) *Svoboda a lidská práva: Její přirozenoprávní základ*, Praha: Vyšehrad.

Sparrow, R. (2014) Ethics, Eugenics, and Politics, in Akabayashi, A. (Ed) *The Future of Bioethics: International Dialogues*, Oxford: Oxford University Press, 139–153.

Sýkora, P. (2014) Kritika teologicko-teleologickej koncepcie ľudskej prirodzenosti ako dôvodu odmietnutia transhumanizmu, *Filozofia* 69 (6), 514–525.

Tomasello, M. (2016) *A Natural History of Human Morality*, Harvard: Harvard University Press.

Chapter 8

Attitudes to progressive gene therapies in Slovakia in the light of the ethical dimensions of human enhancement

Gabriel Bianchi

Abstract: The chapter attempts to bring more understanding into the diversity and dynamics of attitudes to progressive therapies within the broader ethical context of human enhancement. Results from the empirical study in Slovakia are discussed within the frameworks of diverse ethical dimensions of human enhancement (F. Allhoff), ethno-epistemic assemblages as well as of scientific citizenship (A. Irwin, M. Michael). The study (a qualitative exploration in twelve focus group discussions) was comparing attitudes to three different levels of gene therapy (gene scan, somatic gene therapy and germline gene therapy) in general public and in patients with experience of implants and other progressive therapies. The results confirm previous findings of a decreasing support with the increasing technical and ethical requirements of the particular level of gene therapy. A surprising effect was, however, found: personal/bodily experience with progressive therapy may facilitate more positive attitudes and acceptance of the higher-level therapies, while making people more cautious towards the lover levels of gene therapy. The chapter points to a need for transcendence of negativism and affirmative approach to human enhancement challenges (R. Braidotti).

Introduction

"Man is the only creature that refuses to be what he is" (Camus, 1951, p.11). Since the early beginnings of human evolution, we homo sapiens have permanently transcended the limits of our ability. Whether we are talking about fire, the wheel, navigation, electricity or computers, the final outcome is always the enhancement of our intellectual capacities. Recently enhancement has become the focus of attention. Ethical thinking is no longer simply concerned with technological progression, but is becoming a guiding force for technological development. This chapter is an attempt to gain greater understanding of the diversity and changing nature of attitudes to progressive gene therapies - a leading platform of technological advancement - in relation to the ethics of human enhancement and the perennial debate on the slippery-slope argument.

Ethical dimensions

One of the many definitions of human enhancement is that by Roduit et al. (2015): "human enhancement is an intervention in the human body by biotechnological means to *improve* – from some perspective, in some regard, and in a certain domain – the condition of an individual". But we are then immediately confronted with the question of how this *improvement* can be assessed. Based on the *status quo ante* (a relativist backward-looking view) or as an ideal human condition to be achieved through improvement (a normative forward-looking view)? These imply different ethical assessments, that different criteria would be required to legitimize enhancement and progressive gene therapy, especially germline gene therapy. Roduit et al. analyse both these seemingly conflicting/disjunctive approaches and end up accepting a comprehensive approach in which both play an essential role. Roduit et al. demonstrate how the relativist approach is always influenced by a particular normative load and how the normative/ideal approach always contains elements of relativism. Therefore, in order for there to be a productive ethical debate on what should be permitted and recommended in human enhancement and progressive gene therapies, and on what counts as *improvement*, there must first be a comprehensive ethical discussion.

Fritz Allhoff et al. (2011) divide the ethical contexts of human enhancement into six areas, which could serve as the framework for a comprehensive ethical discussion: (1) freedom and autonomy, (2) fairness and equity, (3) social disruptions, (4) human dignity and the good life, (5) rights and obligations and (6) policy and law. They also highlight the importance of the historical/societal context of the moral status of enhancement. Each area of moral assessment is context dependent. If social structures, for example, adapt to accommodate diversity in a specific trait, the enhancement-enabled differences in this trait will lose their moral dimension (if separate competitions were created for enhanced and unenhanced individuals, steroid use in sports might no longer be an ethical issue). Thus once social structures have adapted to account for them, cognitive enhancement or germline gene therapy will no longer be as controversial as they are now.

There is one concept that is fully relevant to the values and the ethical and legal dimensions of the rapid and radical scientific-technological developments in genomic engineering and gene therapy. Paradoxically, it is not based on a value, ethical matter or legal act. It is the slippery slope argument, which holds that adaptive processes, human development and cultural evolution will inevitably progress. The slippery-slope argument has traditionally been linked to moral relativism and weak "will". It is used in relation to the progression of gene technology as a universal label for negative, unwanted development. In the mid-1990s, David Resnik (1994, 1997) used the phenomenon of gene therapy, and specifically of human germline gene therapy, then a mere possibility, "to undermine the slippery slope argument against human germ-line gene therapy (HGLGT) on the grounds that the downside of this slope, genetic enhancement, need not be as immoral or unjust as many people think. Regarding questions of morality, HGLGT's harms to future generations probably will not be as severe as some people imagine, and we can use education to counteract these harms" (Resnik, 1994). The most serious problem Resnik identifies is that of social justice. "HGLGT could lead to grave social injustices and we must take appropriate steps to prevent these consequences if we are to permit its use" (Resnik, 1994). This concern was further elaborated by Resnik in his Rawlsian perspective (Resnik, 1997), in which he concluded that the theory of distributive justice "would allow for genetic inequalities among individuals so long as those inequalities are (a) to everyone's advantage and (b) do not undermine fair equality of opportunity or equality of liberty." Resnik admits that such an approach would need to be informed by a concept of "genetic normality" that defined an adequate range of genetic differences - setting limits on both the upper and the lower bounds of genetic variation so that genetic differences are to everyone's mutual advantage.

Just a few years later, in 2004, Francoise Baylis and Jason Scott Robert published their defence of the inevitability of genetic enhancement technologies. They developed an inevitability thesis: "By 'inevitability' we do not mean to invoke either a technological imperative or a slippery slope, but rather something more akin to 'resilient to (moral) argument and resultant from particular conceptions of contemporary humanity'... to develop and use genetic enhancement technologies are inevitable, not simply because of capitalist forces, heedless liberalism, a natural desire for knowledge or because of a natural or fostered desire to outperform, but also because this is our destiny chosen by those among us who are intent on achieving self-actualisation by controlling the human evolutionary story" (Baylis, Robert, 2004).

Voices warning of the slippery slope continue to be heard; Darnovsky (2013) is a recent example. These are often based on a systematic analysis of the slippery slope phenomenon and the several dimensions (empirical, conceptual and arbitrary; conf. Launis, 2002) relating to it. David Baltimore et al. state that, in the current epoch of the guaranteed safety and efficacy of the technology, concerns about the slippery slope, ranging from disease-curing applications towards those with less compelling or troubling implications, are (merely) one key element in the discussions over whether treating serious human diseases would represent a responsible use of genome engineering, and if so, under what circumstances. For example, would it be appropriate to use the technology to alter a disease-causing genetic mutation to reflect the sequence more typically found in healthy people? Baltimore et al. (2015) are optimistic and outline four recommendations on the steps to be taken to ensure genomic engineering and germline gene modification follow a "prudent path" (*"...steps to take toward ensuring that the application of genome engineering technology is performed safely and ethically."*): (1) strongly discourage any attempts at germline genome modification for clinical application in humans while the societal, environmental and ethical implications are still being discussed by scientific and governmental organizations. This will allow for the identification of any pathways to responsible uses of this technology; (2) create forums in which experts from the scientific and bioethics communities can provide information and training on this new era of human biology and the issues accompanying the risks and rewards of using it; (3) encourage and support transparent research to evaluate the efficacy of CRISPR-Cas9 genome engineering technology and (4) convene a globally representative group, consisting of developers and users of genome engineering technology and experts in genetics, law and bioethics, as well as members of the scientific community, the public and relevant government agencies and interest groups.

Scientific citizenship

The above primarily concerns the expert arena. The public arena, however, comprises multiple stakeholders with their own opinions, attitudes and moral judgements on gene therapy. Rachel Iredale et al. (2003) conducted a pilot qualitative study involving patients with cystic fibrosis and discovered that attitudes on the acceptability of human gene therapy were not necessarily determined by experience of, or exposure to, a genetic condition when compared with students attending science evening classes and lay members of the public. In another early study on moral opinions concerning somatic gene therapy, Scully et al. (2004) found important differences between various groups of patients and particularly between patients and medical professionals. In their qualitative research, they identified eleven major themes concerning the ethics of somatic gene therapy. These were: (1) body and identity, (2) disability and identity, (3) role of genes, (4) eugenics and intolerance, (5) risk and unpredictability, (6) timescale and the life course, (7) financial issues, (8) emotional factors, (9) powerlessness, (10) trust/mistrust and (11) information. The differences in the findings between the various patient groups were important: somatic gene therapy was viewed most positively by multiple sclerosis patients, followed by cystic fibrosis, deaf and achondroplastic patients. However, the most striking differences were found between the patients and the medical professionals. These two groups formulated a different set of arguments each. The medical professionals' set of ethical judgements (1) focused on acceptability based on a strong therapeutic imperative, (2) was based on an unproblematic distinction between identity and disability/illness, and (3) did not consider SGT to be ethically different from other medical interventions. The patients' moral evaluations (1) often questioned the need for, or effectiveness of, "therapeutic" interventions, (2) strongly associated identity with disability/illness and (3) saw genetic interventions as identity altering.

Given the variety of public opinions, the concept of scientific citizenship introduced by Irwin (2001) is relevant to the gene therapy debate. Scientific citizenship involves the construction of publics of citizens who have a legitimate role in the governance of science. It reflects an awareness of the links between science and society and implies that scientific knowledge is not only important for citizenship in contemporary society, but also that citizens can lay legitimate claim to ensuring accountability in scientific research. Scientific citizenship can be perceived as a normative ideal concerning the appropriate form of democratic governance in a society that has become increasingly dependent on scientific knowledge. However, it also requires scientific citizenship to be constructed. The difference between an expert audience and a lay audience, or between science and society, must be grasped before scientific citizenship can be considered, and Irwin and Michael (2003, 108) suggest *ethno-epistemic assemblage*[1] or

[1] Ethno-epistemic assemblage employs Deleuze and Guatarri's concept of assemblage. An assemblage is a representation of multiplicity and heterogeneity, a non-hierarchical, fluid network of disparate objects and associations – it is "rhizomatic" (Deleuze and Guattari 1987) like a system of roots. Deleuze and Guatarri's philosophy emphasizes the importance of multiplicity and heterogeneity in understanding reality and society. Their psycho-analytical approach suggests that the innate motivation of people and society, their desire, is that of infinite possibility and multiplicity, of constantly becoming something rather than achieving a fixed state. Assemblages are not stable, but fluid and constantly becoming, temporally bounded spaces of associated multiplicity, unified to satisfy desire. As a means of linguistically representing complex societal phenomena, ethno-epistemic assemblages may resemble the discursive approach and the textuality and tectonics of discourses (Curt, 1994). The discursive resources approach (Willig, 1993, p. 384) highlights the agency, position and construction of the subjectivity of a subject involved in and exploiting any discourse. The ethno-epistemic assemblage approach is distinct from the platform of discourses, narratives and/or scripts; it is more dynamic, highlighting individual expectations of the future and thus has fruitful analytical implications for the study of publics.

rather conflicting ethno-epistemic assemblages be used for this purpose. An ethno-epistemic assemblage (EEA) is a construct that combines the individual's context (ethnos) and the forms of knowledge relevant to their contexts (episteme) in assemblages, highlighting the interwoven, dynamic and fluid nature of (a specific) episteme against and in conjunction with other EEAs and social narratives (Lee, 2015). Thus it encompasses cognitive, emotional and ethical dimensions. Maja Horst (2007) investigated EEAs in her analysis of a Danish newspaper debate on the experimental use of somatic gene therapy on the liver in Denmark in 1999 in research that had to be prematurely suspended due to "irregularities". Horst identified three EEAs in which medical science, patients, expectations and the governance of science and publics all differed. The first assemblage of consumption concerns patients' rights relating to the production of goods in the form of medical knowledge and treatments; and the need for patients' rights - consumer rights - to be protected in legislation. The second, assemblage of comportment, concerns physicians' responsibilities, and affects the relationships between scientists and other actors through the one-way dissemination of knowledge; they all have to behave according to their prescribed roles and obligations. The third assemblage of heroic action - the "last hope" construct - concerns patients who can only rely on the hope they might encounter an action hero capable of offering them a last chance, since medical science is not expected to produce anything of value. In each of the assemblages, expectations play a different role. In the first assemblage the expectations of future cures are relatively unproblematic and not subjected to questioning. However, in the second assemblage expectations play a crucial role, which, if false or based on unrealistic hopes, may jeopardize the scientific quest for a cure. And in the third assemblage the expectations concern "last hope" solutions - the "heroic action" - rather than systematic scientific efforts. Regardless of these differences in expectation, all three assemblages contain an ethical dimension that is relevant to each of the performative forms of the particular assemblages - the consumption of a progressive cure, the regulated provision of a cure and the non-normative heroic action.

Assessment in Slovakia

The aim of the study was to establish the extent to which progressive gene therapies were approved of in Slovakia by performing qualitative research aimed at exploring the ethical dimensions of human enhancement discussed above (Allhoff et al., 2011) and at considering these in relation to ethno-epistemic assemblages (Horst, 2007) and other relevant conceptual frameworks. We were also interested in two particular quantitative aspects. The first involved comparisons of the three ethically "graduated" forms of gene therapy: gene scanning, somatic gene therapy and germline gene therapy. The research question investigated was: What is the relationship between the increasing significance of the therapies and the extent of approval? The second involved comparing the general population with people who had implants or who had undergone specialist medical treatment. The research question was: Is personal experience of progressive medical technologies related to attitudes to gene therapy?

Method

The empirical study consisted of qualitative research performed in twelve focus group discussions on attitudes to three different levels of gene therapy - gene scanning, somatic gene therapy and germline gene therapy. The focus groups were composed of adults from the general population (8 groups) and patients who had experience of implants and other progressive therapies (4 groups), a total of over 60 participants. The groups were deliberately formed of persons of different age (20–30 and 40–50 years), education (low and higher) and regions from Slovakia, as well as gender balanced, in order to encourage lively discussion. The topics discussed were: (1) A vignette narrative about Angelina Jolie to stimulate discussion on choosing to undergo mastectomy-based gene scanning medical advice, (2) Opinions on gene scanning therapy (Therapy1), (3) Opinions on somatic gene therapy (Therapy 2) and (4) Opinions on germline gene therapy (Therapy 3). The discussion was facilitated by an experienced psychologist, recorded and fully transcribed.

Analysis

The various arguments in favour of and/or against the types of gene therapy were open coded according to the conceptual areas they exploited and - where possible - were organized using the six categories of ethical arguments formulated by Allhof et al. (2011) - **Freedom and Autonomy,**

Fairness and Equity, Social Disruptions, Human Dignity and the Good Life, Rights and Obligations, Policy and Law. The focus group discussions were then quantitatively analysed, with the arguments in favour of and against each type of gene therapy being counted separately for each focus group. On the basis of these figures, the differences were analysed for comparative purposes according to (1) approval of the three types of gene therapy and (2) differences between the general population and patients with implants or experience of progressive therapies. Finally the arguments used were subjected to a qualitative analysis.

Results

The quantitative analysis of attitudes to gene therapy showed that there is general approval of this sensitive issue. However, there are important differences in the extent of approval the Slovak participants accorded to the three different therapies, with "simplest" and most accessible option of gene scanning achieving the highest level of approval (the index of approval was 20.2, meaning there were 20 times as many "pro" voices than voices "against"). Paradoxically, however, the gene scanning in the vignette situation that drew on a decision recommended on the basis of a gene scan (Angelina Jolie's voluntary mastectomy) was seen as least acceptable to the participants, with most statements rejecting her decision (index of approval 0.56). The somatic and germline gene therapies were both regarded with approval overall, but at a significantly lower level than the gene scanning. The indices of approval for these therapies were 2.45 and 3.57, respectively, indicating similar support to public opinion. Table 1 shows these differences.

However, when participants' experiences are taken into account, these clearly have an effect on the extent to which particular types of gene therapy are approved of. When compared to participants from the general population, participants with implants and/or experience of advanced therapies do not manifest the same high level of support for gene scanning, and they approved less of Angelina Jolie's decision; at the same time, however, they have more positive attitudes to somatic and germline therapy (see Table 2).

The quantitative analysis of support/rejection for each progressive therapy is accompanied by **qualitative analysis**. This enables us to assess

Table 1: Index of approval of gene therapies: (Figures >1 indicate approval and the number of times the pro statements exceeded the against statements; figures <1 indicate rejection and the proportion of pro statements to against statements)

(Approval/ Rejection)	F1 20–30BA	F2 40–50 BA	F3 High Edu BA	F4 Low Edu BA	F5 20–30 MT	F6 40–50 MT	F7 High Edu ZA	F8 Low Edu ZA	F9 Impl etc BA	F10 Impl etc BA	F11 Impl etc MT	F12 Impl etc ZA	TOTAL
Angelina Jolie/ Gene Scan	3.5:2.5	3:3	1:5	3.5:2.5	2.5:3.5	1:4	1:4	2:4	1:4	2:2	2:2	0:4	22.5:40.5 = 0.56
THERAPY 1 Gene Scanning	6:0	5.5:0.5	5:0	6:0	6:0	5.5:0.5	4:0	5:0	1.5:0.5	1:0	3:0	2:1	50.5:2.5 = 20.2
THERAPY 2 Somatic	2:3	3.5:0.5	4:2	1.5:2.5	5:0	4:2	1:1	3.5:0.5	2.5:0.5	2.5:0.5	4:0	2:2	35.5:14.5 = 2.45
THERAPY 3 Germline	5:0	5:0	3:2	1:1	2:3	4.5:1.5	3:0	4:1	3:0	2.5:0.5	2.5:1.5	2:0	37.5:10.5 = 3.57

Note: Groups can be identified by age, education and region of participants (BA=Bratislava, ZA=Žilina, MT=Martin). Groups with participants with experience of implants or other progressive therapies are identified with „Impl etc".

Table 2: Index of approval of gene therapies – participants with implants vs. general population: (Figures >1 indicate approval and the number of times the pro statements exceeded the against statements; figures <1 indicate rejection and the proportion of pro statements to against statements)

(Y/N)	F1 20–30 BA	F2 40–50 BA	F3 High Edu BA	F4 Low Edu BA	F5 20–30 MT	F6 40–50 MT	F7 High Edu ZA	F8 Low Edu ZA	NO IM-PLANTS:	F9 Impl etc BA	F10 Impl etc BA	F11 Impl etc MT	F12 Impl etc ZA	IM-PLANTS:
Angelina Gene Scan	3.5:2.5	3:3	1:5	3.5:2.5	2.5:3.5	1:4	1:4	2:4	17.5:28.5 = 0.61	1:4	2:2	2:2	0:4	5:12 = 0.42
THER 1 Gene Scanning	6:0	5.5:0.5	5:0	6:0	6:0	5.5:0.5	4:0	5:0	43:1 = 43	1.5:0.5	1:0	3:0	2:1	7.5:1.5 = 5
THER 2 Somatic	2:3	3.5:0.5	4:2	1.5:2.5	5:0	4:2	1:1	3.5:0.5	24.5:11.5 = 2.13	2.5:0.5	2.5:0.5	4:0	2:2	11:3 = 3.67
THER 3 Germline	5:0	5:0	3:2	1:1	2:3	4.5:1.5	3:0	4:1	27.5:8.5 = 3.24	3:0	2.5:0.5	2.5:1.5	2:0	10:2 = 5

Note: Groups can be identified by age, education and region of participants (BA=Bratislava, ZA=Žilina, MT=Martin). Groups with participants with experience of implants or other progressive therapies are identified with „Impl etc".

which moral discourses feature in the public discourses on progressive gene therapies in Slovakia. Of the six ethical contexts Allhoff et al. (2011) describe that can be used to frame discourses on human enhancement three could be identified in the discussions: **Freedom and Autonomy, Fairness and Equity, Human Dignity and the Good Life.** Another seven categories also emerged: **Probability vs. Causality, Distrust – Authority, Relativism – Slippery Slope, Religion, Scepticism, Fear and Managing unknowns – human and environmental concerns and long-term effects**. The ethical context categories suggested by Allhoff et al. (2011) which we could not identify were Social Disruptions, Rights and Obligations and Policy and Law (see Table 3).

Table 3: Arguments made by participants in the focus group discussions by category of ethical relevance

Topic	Category of ethical argument	Attitude	Argument (direct quotations in italics)
ANGELINA/ Gene scan	Fairness and Equity:	AGAINST	• *Who would pay for it?* • NIMBY
	Human Dignity and Good Life:	PRO	• *We should admire Angelina's decision.* • *I agree. I would do the same as long as my husband didn't have a problem with it.* • *Implants are common.* • *You can live a full life with implants.*
	Freedom and Autonomy:	PRO	• Family responsibilities vs. living alone • *I'd rather give up a small bit of my body than lose a big part.* • *Angelina's motive might have been to increase her popularity.*
	Probability vs. Causality:	AGAINST/ PRO	• *The problem hasn't been solved.* • *Cancer can pop up anywhere in the body (later).* • *Probability is not sufficient reason to act.* • *Cancer is curable these days.* • *I would try alternative medicines, a special diet, to prevent genetic predispositions.* • *There is still the possibility you might not get the cancer...* • *There are modern effective treatments for cancer.* • *I have a friend who got cancer and they were able to treat her successfully.* • Doubts about genetic determination – stress is a crucial factor in cancer. • Cognitive-emotional transfer: knowing the risks causes fear. • *It is better to wait till you have symptoms.* • *Prevention is the right way.*

	Distrust – Authority:	AGAINST	• Undergoing mastectomia to be even more fancy • *Maybe it didn't happen at all, maybe it was just a health-promotion advertising trick.* • *Is it an advertising trick for breast implants?* • *All unnecessary surgery is pointless. I could be killed in a car crash at anytime...* • *Surgery might not work* • *Patient-doctor communication has failed* • *Doctors make mistakes* • *Our doctors make the surgery superficially.* • *Cancer can be treated if diagnosed early.* • *I wouldn't do things that trigger cancer but protect myself: the pill, and breastfeeding.* • *In order to decide (you have to) consult a doctor, i.e. someone in authority.*
	Scepticism	PRO/ AGAINST	• *I'm against it out of principle and I believe most people in Slovakia would be against it.*
	Relativism – Slippery Slope	PRO	• *Experiencing the death of a close relative increases one's willingness to accept this "prevention"*
	Fear:	PRO/ AGAINST	• *I would go for it because the fear could trigger the cancer.* • *We shouldn't act/decide in haste, out of fear.*
Gene Scanning	Religion:	PRO	• *Anyone could agree with this – whether they're religious or not.*
	Fairness and Equity:	PRO/ AGAINST	• Selective use for those who "need" it for health reasons • *You can't help everyone.*
	Managing unknowns, human and environmental concerns and long-term effects:	PRO/ AGAINST	• Risk of self-obsession for humankind
	Probability vs. Causality:	AGAINST/ PRO	• *Probability is not causality; you could stay healthy even though the probability is 99%...* • *This is mainly about serious diseases like cancer.*
	Dis/trust vs. Authority:	MAINLY AGAINST	• Paranoia about the healthcare system and the pharma industry ("they don't want us to get better") • *The pharma industry intentionally keeps people sick.* • Pharma lobby – medicines contain triggers for other diseases • *Science should focus on preventing diseases.* • *Sometimes patient regulate the dosage more precisely...*

	Dis/trust vs. Authority:	MAINLY AGAINST	• *You can't trust anyone today, but we should trust our doctor.* • *Consult another doctor (=authority) before deciding; not the internet.*
Somatic Gene Therapy	Religion:	PRO	• *Religion is not a barrier (for me).* • *This could cause a problem for religious people, but there's no ethical issue here for me.* • *In spite of the religious arguments, this issue has nothing to do with playing God.*
	Fairness and Equity:	NOT AGAINST	Will not be accessible to all people because of cost
	Managing unknowns, human and environmental concerns and long-term effects:	AGAINST	• Risk of negative side effects • Fear of side effects • *This could change the nature of man.* • *When treating one organ, another could fail.* • *You might turn into a monster.* • *It's like experimenting on rabbits – who knows whether the body will accept it.* • *OK, unless there are side effects.*
	Fear:	NOT AGAINST	• The stem/germ cells would need to come from a relative, not an unknown person
Germline gene therapy	Religion:	PRO	• *I'm religious and would have no problem with it – it's my health and my child and that's what's important to me; I don't care what others say.*
	Fairness and Equity:	AGAINST	• *This could create an "enhanced oligarchy" of rich people who can afford the therapy*
	Human Dignity and Good Life:	AGAINST	• *I have a sick child and it's no problem for me.* • *Having perfect children is not a guarantee of happiness.* • *Why should anyone correct something that has existed for generations – our blood line.* • Some participants concentrate most on themselves, their disease and treatment failures, and do not really consider germ-transfer
	Freedom and Autonomy:	PRO	• *I would agree and volunteer for experiments.* • *I am for progress, willing to participate in experiments using new therapies.* • *I would agree even if there was some (small) potential risk.*

	Managing unknowns, human and environmental concerns and long-term effects:	MAINLY AGAINST	• *This therapy crosses over the line into human enhancement; how/who will determine whether it is just therapy or enhancement?* • *I fear this would lead to abuse (e.g. eugenics).* • Risk of abuse of human enhancement – producing mass murderers, etc. • Fear of uncertainty about future advances. • *Will we soon we have a "perfect human", a robot?* • *It's OK for treatment purposes, but not to make the human body into a machine, at a certain moment, before "perfection" is reached, it needs to be stopped.* • *Earth's population will increase.* • Unavoidable (unknown) "consequences" • *"If there are no serious (additional) risks."* • The triggering of negative effects??? • *New diseases might be "created".* • Conditional agreement – if unwanted effects could be prevented • Other negative consequences may arise. • Risk of unexpected consequences
	Probability vs. Causality and Scepticism:	SELECTIVE and SCEPTIC PRO	• *How serious is the disease in question?* • *This should only be used in relation to fatal, serious diseases.* • *I could agree with it if the disease was fatal, serious.* • *Be careful; nature is more complex than we think.* • *New diseases will emerge anyhow...*

Below is a table showing the ten ethical context categories divided into the four therapies they were explored in relation to. It shows support, rejection or ambivalence for the gene therapy in relation to each ethical context (see Table 4).

Table 4: Reference to gene therapy in relation to ethical context

Ethical context:	Type of gene therapy:	PRO	PRO/against ambivalence	Against
Freedom and Autonomy	Angelina	x		
	Gene Scanning			
	Somatic Gene therapy			
	Germline Gene therapy		x	
Fairness and Equity	Angelina			x
	Gene Scanning		x	
	Somatic Gene therapy		x	
	Germline Gene therapy			x
Human Dignity and Good Life	Angelina	x		
	Gene Scanning			
	Somatic Gene therapy			
	Germline Gene therapy			x
Probability vs. Causality	Angelina		x	
	Gene Scanning		x	
	Somatic Gene therapy			
	Germline Gene therapy		x	
Distrust – Authority	Angelina			x
	Gene Scanning			x
	Somatic Gene therapy			
	Germline Gene therapy			
Relativism – Slippery slope	Angelina	x		
	Gene Scanning			
	Somatic Gene therapy			
	Germline Gene therapy			
Religiosity	Angelina			
	Gene Scanning	x		
	Somatic Gene therapy	x		
	Germline Gene therapy	x		
Scepticism	Angelina		x	
	Gene Scanning			
	Somatic Gene therapy			
	Germ-line Gene therapy			
Fear	Angelina		x	
	Gene Scanning			
	Somatic Gene therapy		x	
	Germline Gene therapy			
Managing unknowns	Angelina			
	Gene Scanning		x	
	Somatic Gene therapy			x
	Germline Gene therapy			x

It is clear from Table 4 that there is no unambiguous position in most of the ethical context categories. The arguments that fed into these categories were frequently "undecided", or came from both sides. The exceptions are *Authority* (linked to Distrust), where only arguments against the use of gene therapy were made (e.g. "*Doctors make mistakes*"), *Religion*, where all the arguments were in support of gene therapy (surprisingly) ("*I'm religious and would have no problem with it – it is MY health and MY child and that's what's important to me; I don't care what others say*") and *Relativism – Slippery Slope*, where the arguments were in support of gene therapies („*Experiencing the death of a close relative increases one's willingness to accept this 'prevention'*").

Conclusions

The analysis of this pilot study has produced several surprising findings. The first is that among Slovak participants there is general significant support for any form of gene therapy presented as a medical challenge, extremely high support for gene scanning and much lower, but still clear, support for somatic gene therapy and germline gene therapy. However, when gene therapy was presented as a VIP-related "case" narrative, even the simplest therapy, gene scanning, was rejected by the majority.

The second surprising finding is the attitude of those already undergoing technology-based treatment and progressive treatment to compensate for disabilities. These participants showed an "inverted" attitude, that is, much lower support for "simple" gene scanning, which could be interpreted as a form of "radical prevention". On the other hand, they were far more approving of the use of progressive somatic and germline gene therapies than participants from the general population. These findings contrast to those of Scully (2004), who found that when patients morally evaluated the use of somatic gene therapy they often questioned the need for, or effectiveness of, "therapeutic" interventions. If we consider the differences between the patients and the participants from the general population in relation to the potential for scientific citizenship (Irwin, 2001), their ethno-epistemic assemblages on progressive gene therapies resemble the distinctions between the ethno-epistemic assemblages on progressive gene therapies identified by Horst (2007). The *assemblage of consumption* (consumption of therapy) can be seen as most relevant to the patients in our pilot study given their positive and relatively unproblematic expectations regarding future treatments; these expectations were not questioned to any substantial degree. The *assemblage of comportment*

(comportment of clear, unequivocal scientific knowledge) could be related to the general population participants, since their expectations related to "scientific proof" and whether insufficient or unrealistic arguments had been raised, and this could limit their approval (and jeopardize the scientific quest for a cure).

The third surprising issue concerns the ethical arguments used in the discussions. Resnik (1997) found that social justice was the most challenging dimension of moral assessment on human enhancement. While Fairness and Equity was more important in Allhoff (2011). Our data indicate that fairness received greater emphasis. Fairness and Equity appeared in the discussions on all the gene therapies. The arguments either belonged to the "undecided" category or to both sides. However, Fairness and Equity was only one of nine categories that appeared during the discussions, and Authority/Distrust, Probability/Causality, Managing unknowns and Human dignity and Good life contained the most varied arguments - all tended towards the "rejection" side in the arguments against gene therapies. The positive arguments approving gene therapies were less elaborate (Autonomy, Religiosity and Slippery-slope) and so one would expect agency in support of these progressive therapies to be relatively low. Resnik's early expectation (1994, 1997) that HGLGT could lead to grave social injustices if genetic inequalities were allowed among individuals, so long as they were to everyone's advantage and did not undermine equal opportunity or equal liberty, now seems too optimistic even twenty years later.

The complexity of ethical thinking on human enhancement and gene therapies, which represent a tiny part of the posthuman transition, is captured in Rosi Braidotti's statement that in posthuman ethics the key notion is "the transcendence of negativity... the conditions for renewed political and ethical agency cannot be drawn from the current state of the terrain. They have to be generated affirmatively and creatively by efforts geared to creating possible futures, by mobilizing resources and visions that have been left untapped and by actualizing them in daily practices of interconnections with others" (Braidotti, 2013, 191). In light of this the broad spectrum of arguments that emerged in the group discussion may be seen to reflect the daily practices of interconnected people continuously constructing their scientific citizenship. This also reflects the ongoing debate on the slippery slope dilemma - to cope with the ethical dimensions of gene therapies we need to follow a "prudent path", allowing them to be used on humans and then we can thoroughly analyse their affirmative values.

Acknowledgement

This work was supported by Slovak Research and Development Agency contract No. APVV-0379-12.

Literature

Allhoff, F., Lin, P., Steinberg, J. (2011) Ethics of human enhancement: An executive summary, *Science and Engineering Ethics*, 17, pp. 201–212.

Baltimore, D., Berg, P., Botchan, M., Carroll, D., et al.(2015) A prudent path forward for genomic engineering and germline gene modification, Science, 348(6230):36

Baylis, F., Robert, J.S. (2004) The inevitability of genetic enhancement technologies, *Bioethics,* 18: 1–26.

Braidotti, R. (2013) *The Posthuman*. Cambridge, Polity.

Camus, A (1951) L´homme révolté. Paris, Gallimard.

Curt, B. C. (1994) Textuality and Tectonics. London, Open University Press.

Daley, G.Q., Doudna, J.A., Fenner, M., Greely, H.T., Jinek, M. Martin, G.S. Enhoet, E., Puck, J., Sternberg, S.H., Eissman, J.S., Yamamoto, K.R. (2015) A prudent path forward for genomic engineering and germline gene modification, *Science*, 348(6230): 36–8.10.1126/science.aab1028

Darnovsky, M.A. (2013) A slippery slope to human germline modification, *Nature*, 499: 127.

Deleuze, G., Guattari, F. (1987) A Thousand Plateaus. Minneapolis: University of Minnesota Press.

Horst, M. (2007) Public expectations of gene therapy: Scientific futures and their performative effects on scientific citizenship, *Science, Technology, and Human Values*, 32: 150–171.

Iredale, R., Dolan, G., McDonald, K., Kirk, M. (2003) Public attitudes to human gene therapy: A pilot study in Wales, *Community Genetics*, 6: 139–146.

Irwin, A. (2001) Constructing the scientific citizen: Science and democracy in the biosciences, *Public understanding of Science*, 10: 1–18.

Irwin, A., Michael, M. (2003) *Science, social theory and public knowledge*. Maidenhead, UK, Open University Press.

Launis, V (2002) Human gene therapy and the slippery slope argument, *Medicine, Health Care and Philosophy*, 5: 169–172.

Lee, A. (2015) Integrating subjects: Linking surveillance experiences to social patterns using ethno-epistemic assemblages, *Surveillance and Society*, 13: 385–399.

Resnik, D. (1994) Debunking the slippery slope argument against human germline gene therapy, *The Journal of Medicine and Philosophy*, 19: 23–40.

Resnik, D. (1997) Genetic engineering: A Rawlsian approach, *Social Theory and Practice*, 23, 427–448.

Roduit, J.A.R., Baumann, H., Heilinger, J.-C. (2014) Evaluating human enhancements: the importance of ideals. *Monash Bioethics Review*, 32: 205–216.

Scully, J.L., Rippberger, C., Rehmann-Sutter, C., (2004) Non-professionals' evaluation of gene therapy ethics, *Social Science and Medicine*, 58: 1415–1425.

Willig, C. (1993) *Introducing Qualitative Research in Psychology*. Berkshire, McGraw-Hill.

Chapter 9

The surgeon's failure to enhance and tort liability. Polish civil law perspective

Andrzej Girdwoyń and Joanna Różyńska

Abstract: The use of cognitive enhancement technologies raises not only ethical, but also legal questions. Numerous scholars have expressed concerns that these technologies may pose a threat to basic human rights, especially the individual's right to self-determination. In response to this worry, the concept of "cognitive liberty" (as a right to be and not to be subjected to enhancing procedures) has been introduced. Many commentators have wondered how cognitive enhancement interventions would change basic concepts and principles of criminal law and criminal responsibility. Yet, little attention has been given so far to the implications of cognitive enhancement technologies for the civil law domain. The aim of this paper is to fill this gap. First we remind the basic tenants of the continental law doctrine on civil liability through the perceptive of the German, French, and Polish legal systems. Second, we identify main challenges the use of cognitive enhancement technologies poses for civil liability. We analyse three elements justifying a claim for damages, namely unlawful conduct of an agent, damage, and causation. We focus on the first and the third one. Regarding the first element, we discuss the problem of agency of a cognitively enhanced individual, especially the influence of his or her enhanced cognition on the standard of *due care* and - what follows - conception of negligence. As to the third element, we analyse the causal relationship between the fact of an enhancement and the damages caused by the enhanced agent. We illustrate these theoretical inquiries with an example of a surgeon who performs a complicated operation under the influence of 200mg of modafinil. In the last part of the paper, we offer some general comments on possible developments of civil law in the era of cognitive enhancement technologies.

Introduction

A growing body of research suggests that some pharmacological substances, such as modafinil and methylphenidate, originally developed to treat neurological or psychiatric conditions, may significantly improve some aspects of cognitive performance in healthy individuals. However, the use of such substances for cognitive enhancement raises not only safety concerns, but also numerous ethical, social, and economic controversies (Bostrom and Sandberg 2009; Sandberg 2011; Sandberg and Savulescu 2011; Housden, Morein-Zamir and Sahakian 2011; Bostrom and Roache 2011, Hildt and Franke 2013; Jotterand and Dubljevic 2016). Recently, it has also attracted attention of legal scholars, who have been debating whether there is a legal obligation for representatives of professions prone to fatigue-related errors due to long work hours, such as pilots or surgeons, to enhance themselves, and if yes, whether a professional, who would refuse to self-enhance, could be liable for negligence for a resulted damage (Vincent 2011, 2013; Chandler 2013; de Sio, Faulmüller and Vincent 2014; Goold and Maslen 2015). The last problem has been extensively examined by scholars from University of Oxford, Imogen Goold and Hannah Maslen (2014a; 2014b).

Goold and Maslen discuss a fictional case of a surgeon, who failed to use modafinil - a eugeroic substance, increasing levels of wakefulness and mental vigilance in individuals who are sleep deprived - and committed a mistake during a medical procedure. Their analyses are based on and limited to English law of tort and the English case law. They focus on the negligence and the scope of the surgeon's duty of care, as well as on the causal link between the physician's omission to enhance and the damage suffered by the patient. Goold and Maslen conclude that:

> "it is highly unlikely that any English court will find that a surgeon (or other professional) who fails to self-enhance and then causes harm will be in breach of her duty to care. But if we are wrong, and such a step is taken, the current capacity of enhancing drugs and devices, and the nature of the capacities they affect, will present difficult challenges regarding causation that any such claims are still likely to fall". (2014b, 453)

The aim of this article is to determine whether the case presented by Goold and Maslen would be decided differently if analysed through the lenses of continental European civil law system, namely the Polish tort law. Our analysis consists of four parts. First, we briefly review current methods of cognitive enhancement, their nature, and effectiveness. Following the Oxford scholars, we concentrate on modafinil as the most promising pharmacological cognitive enhancer. Second, we introduce the case of surgeon Jane, as described by Goold and Maslen. Third, we present basic concepts and conditions of civil liability under the Polish tort law. Finally, we apply principles of the Polish tort law to the Jane's case. We conclude that also in the Polish tort law claims in negligence against medical professionals for injuries, allegedly caused by a failure to use cognitive enhancers, are unlikely to succeed.

1. Cognitive enhancers – an overview

Cognitive enhancement, in the broadest sense, means any intervention used with the intent to improve human cognitive capacities beyond their normal range (Bostrom and Sandberg 2009; Sandberg 2011). Such improvement may be achieved by various methods - from using illegal drugs to taking a walk in a park. In this paper we focus only on biomedical means of cognitive enhancement, which in turn can be divided into two categories: non-pharmacological and pharmacological. The non-pharmacological methods include transcranial magnetic stimulation, TMS (Klimesch, Sauseng and Gerloff 2003; Zimerman and Hummel 2010), transcranial direct-current stimulation, tDCS (Coffman, Clark and Parasuraman 2014; Richmond et al. 2014), and brain-machine interfaces (Vlek et al. 2012). Although available scientific data suggest certain level of efficiency of these methods, following Goold and Maslen, we will pay special attention to pharmacological cognitive enhancers. The authors rightly point out that a failure to take psychopharmacological substances is the most likely source of a claim in negligence against medical professionals (2014b, 430).

In the category of pharmacological methods of cognitive enhancement, three subgroups may be distinguished based on the criterion of their legal accessibility: illegal substances, legal dietary products and dietary supplements, and legally registered medical products (drugs). Our analysis includes neither illegal enhancement substances, such as for example amphetamine, nor legal dietary supplements such as caffeinated drinks or ginkgo biloba. We focus only on the off-label use of legal, prescription drugs, in particular drugs with the most popular substance used to combat fatigue - modafinil.

Modafinil is a drug registered in numerous countries under different trade names, such as 'Vigil', 'Provigil', 'Modasomil', 'Modiodal', or 'Alertec' (U.S. FDA 1998; EMA 2010). It is a wakefulness-promoting agent approved for therapy of excessive sleepiness associated with chronic diseases, such as narcolepsy or shift work sleep disorder. However, studies have shown that when used by healthy individuals, both fatigued or not-sleep deprived, modafinil demonstrates certain nootropic effects. It improves visual attention, reaction time, psychomotor speed (Grady et al. 2010; Hart et al. 2006), enhances memory, planning and decision-making (Müller et al. 2013), and selectively improves neuropsychological task performance (Turner et al. 2003). Also research involving sleep-deprived pilots and physicians have provided some evidence that modafinil decreases feeling of depression and anger; improves vigour, alertness, and confidence (Caldwell et al. 2004, Caldwell 2005); improves attention, cognitive control, and working memory of fatigued professionals (Gill et al. 2006); attenuates impulsive and enhances mental processes critical for efficient information processing, flexible thinking, and decision-making under time pressure (Sugden et al. 2012). The research does not, however, provide sufficiently clear and favourable evidence to recommend the use of modafinil in the workplace. The same as well as other studies suggest that modafinil cognitive benefits are much more limited (Turner et al. 2003; Randall et al. 2003; Randall et al. 2005; Müller et al. 2013). And, even if the drug enables professionals to operate on duty longer, it does not have a significant effect on their psychomotor control and performance, beyond very simple tasks, and what follows, on the reduction of fatigue-related errors (Sugden et al. 2012). No doubt, more research is needed both on modafinil safety and ability to improve various cognitive functions in healthy subjects. What seems to be certain is that modafinil cannot replace sleep or proper rest.

2. The scenario

Goold and Maslen provide the following scenario of a surgeon's failure to self-enhance, which will be the basis of our legal analysis as well:

> "A surgeon, Jane, has worked twenty-four hours without sleep. She is about to leave the hospital at the end of her shift when an emergency case arrives. The patient, Richard, needs a complex surgery due to a traumatic brain injury, and the surgeon is the only one who can perform it, as the only other surgeon employed at the hospital who could perform it is busy with another, long surgery. The patient's case is urgent; if he does not receive the operation, his condition will rapidly deteriorate. Jane knows she is exhausted, but thinks she can stay sufficiently alert and competent for the duration of the surgery required, which she expects to be about two hours in length. However, she knows there is a risk that she might make an error due to her fatigued state. She also knows that the only alternative is for the patient to be diverted to the nearest other hospital, which is more than an hour's drive away, which will almost certainly mean his condition will worsen, potentially fatally.

She is seemingly faced with a choice between two options, both of which entail a risk to the patient: perform the surgery while tired (and possibly make an error due to her fatigue) or refuse to accept the patient and insist he is diverted elsewhere (exposing him to the risk that this condition will worsen). However, in our scenario, it is normal practice for Jane and her colleagues at the hospital to use modafinil when fatigued. Jane therefore has a third option: take the modafinil and then perform the surgery, hoping that it will decrease the effects of her fatigue. In our scenario, she chooses to undertake the surgery without taking the modafinil. Richard suffers harm as a result of the surgery and alleges that it occurred because Jane made a fatigue-related error." (2014b, 431–432)

3. Conditions for physician's liability – the Polish law perspective

The Polish civil law system distinguishes two civil liability regimes for damages: *ex delicto* and *ex contractu*. *Ex delicto* liability, also known as tort liability, arises when the damage is caused by a wrongful (faulty) act or omission. *Ex contractu* liability, on the other hand, arises when the damage is a result of the failure to perform, or the improper performance of a previously undertaken contractual obligation. In what follows, we focus only on tort liability for one's own behaviour.

The general clause of tort liability for one's own conduct is expressed in article 415 of the Civil Code of the Republic of Poland of 23rd April 1964 (with further amendments; further referred to as the CC). The provision stipulates that "whoever by his fault causes a damage to another person shall be obliged to redress it". Despite its laconic form, the provision states all conditions for tort liability under the Polish law, namely the existence of damage, faulty conduct, and the causal link between the conduct and the damage (Bagińska and Tulibacka 2014). Let us take a closer look at the last two conditions.

It is considered that the term "fault", used in the article 415 of the CC, covers two elements: a broadly understood objective unlawfulness (wrongfulness, illegality) of a tortfeasor's conduct and his subjective fault (guilt). The objective unlawfulness of a conduct consists in a violation of legal norms, in particular those determining legal duties of the tortfeasor, or in a violation of the so-called rules of social coexistence (Żmij 2009). As far as the conduct of physician towards patients is concerned, article 4 of the Act of the Professions of Physician and Dentist of 5th December 1996 (with further amendments) is of a great importance. The article states that the physician is obliged to perform his professional duties in accordance with the indications of actual medical knowledge, use of available methods and means of preventing, diagnosing, and treating diseases, with adherence to the rules of professional ethics, and with due care and diligence. A violation of any of these requirements makes the physician's act or omission unlawful.

The second component of "fault" of a tortfeasor's conduct is his subjective fault. In theory, the fault may take one of two forms – intentional and unintentional, i.e. negligence. However, in the Polish tort law the distinction between intentional and unintentional conduct does not have much of significance as any departure, even the least, from the standard of due care, makes a tortfeasor liable for negligence and obliged to repair the damage caused. Thus, although the fault of a tortfeasor has been traditionally viewed as a subjective condition for tort liability, it is measured objectively by comparing an actual conduct of the tortfeasor with the model conduct expected in a given situation from a person of a given characteristic.

The standard of due care of a physician is higher than expected from an average person as it takes into account the professional character of his activity (article 355 § 2 of the CC). Physicians are highly trained professionals, and they are expected to treat patients in accordance with the adequate and actual medical knowledge, skills, diligence, and carefulness. Moreover, they operate on human goods of the highest individual and social value, namely health and life, and their breach of the duty of due care may result in a violation of patients' most fundamental rights and interests. In practice, courts dealing with medical malpractice cases establish the applicable standard of due care by comparing the conduct of the physician in question with an abstract "model of a good physician" – a model of a competent, skilful, and diligent physician of a respective medical discipline. The model is objective, but flexible. It is based on standards set by relevant legal norms, principles of medical ethics, professional guidelines, and life experience. It is related not only to medical specialization, but also to level of professional qualification and experience. The model is placed against all relevant circumstances of a given case, especially those beyond the physician's control which might have negatively affected his ability to meet the model's requirements (Kalus 2009; Bączyk-Rozwadowska 2011; Nesterowicz 2013).

The Polish civil law adopts a theory of the so-called adequate causation (Koch 1975). Pursuant to article 361 § 1 of the CC "the person obliged to pay compensation is liable only for the normal effects of the act or omission from which the damage resulted". This principle limits the scope of a tortfeasor's compensatory duty only to injuries, harms, or losses incurred by the damaged party that are usual, ordinary, typical consequences of the tortfeasor's faulty conduct. He is not obliged to pay damages for unusual or extraordinary consequences of his acts or omissions.

In order to establish the scope of the tortfeasor' liability, a two-step test is performed (Koch 1975). The first step involves a *conditio sine qua non* test. The aim of the test is to determine whether the damage would have occurred, if the alleged tortfeasor had not behaved as he in fact did. The test requires an attentive examination of all the specific circumstance of the case at hand. Thus, its result is usually *quaestio facti*. Both the Polish jurisprudence and case law emphasize that the causal link between the tortfeasor's conduct and the damage may be direct or indirect, and it does not have to be certain (Kalus 2009; Bagińska 2011, 2013; Bączyk-Rozwadowska 2011; Nesterowicz 2013). It is enough to show that it is highly probable that without a putative causal factor (tortfeasor's act or omission), the result (damage) would not have happened. Thus, the "high degree of probability" is sufficient for establishing the necessary causation between the delictive conduct and the damage (Bagińska 2011). It is particularly important in medical malpractice cases, since – due to the diversity of human body responses to medical interventions as well as the differences in patterns of a disease development – it is often difficult to identify the causal factor that led to the injury with absolute certainty.

If the *conditio sine qua non* test proves that the tortfeasor's conduct was a necessary condition of the damage, the next step is to decide whether the damage suffered by the victim falls within the rage of normal consequences of such a conduct. The "normality" of the relation between causal factor and the effect is evaluated in the light of current scientific knowledge, life experience, and specific circumstances of the case, including particular characteristics of the victim that could and should be known to the tortfeasor. "Normal" effects of an action are those, "which occurrence in more probable each time a causal factor of a given kind occurs" (Koch 1975, 137). And normal consequences of an omission are those "which occurrence is less probable or impossible each time the [actually abandoned] action is undertaken" (Koch 1975, 151) or – to put it in other words – which probability increases each time the omission in question takes place. In must be stressed that the rise of the probability of the effect does not have to be very high. It must be high enough to justify the claim that whenever a given action or omission takes place, it is – in the light of scientific knowledge and life experience - reasonable to expect that a given effect will happen.

4. Could Jane be found liable under the Polish tort law?

In the scenario, borrowed from Goold and Maslen, Jane - a fatigued surgeon still on a shift - faces three options: (1) to perform a complex and long-lasting brain surgery on new coming emergency patient Richard, without using any kind of cognitive enhancement; (2) to take modafinil, as majority of her hospital colleagues does, and then perform a complex surgery on the patient; (3) to refuse to accept the patient and insist he is diverted elsewhere. She chooses the first option and commits a medical error in result of which Richard suffers harm.

The case is described in very general terms, therefore, for the sake of the accuracy of further legal analysis, three additional comments must be made. First, we assume that Richard brings a compensatory claim against Jane for injuries, which - in his opinion - are the consequence of medical fatigue-related error committed by the surgeon. Second, we assume that the patient does not argue that Jane could and should have prevented the fatigue-related error by referring him to another hospital, but rather that she could and should have prevented the error by using modafinil. And third, we assume that the medical error committed by Jane is negligent. This is an important point, since not every medical error, defined as a deviation from a required standard of due care (from an abstract "model of a good physician") constitutes a negligence. Sometimes a physician's failure to meet the standard is justified or even unavoidable. With all these additional remarks in mind, we may proceed with the case analysis.

4.1. Was Jane's decision "faulty"?

In order to succeed in the Polish civil court, Richard has to prove that:

- By not taking modafinil Jane acted in a "faulty" manner - her omission was unlawful and she was guilty of the omission, at least negligent.
- There is an adequate causal link between the Jane' omission and the damage suffered by Richard in result of the improperly performed surgery.

As mentioned earlier, a physician is liable for an injury caused to his patient only if his harmful conduct was unlawful and guilt based, in particular if it constituted a breach of the physician's duty of due care. Does Jane's decision to abstain from taking modafinil meet these requirements? No. Neither the Polish law nor the Code of Medical Ethics of the Polish physicians, nor any relevant professional guideline require or encourage physicians, who are overworked, to take modafinil to overcome fatigue and sleepiness at work. In fact, modafinil was registered in Poland under the trade name 'Vigil', but the producer withdrew it from the market in 2011 (Torrex Chiesi Polska Sp. z.o.o. 2011). When available, it was approved only for excessive sleepiness associated with chronic diseases in adults, including narcolepsy, obstructive sleep apnea hypopnea syndrome, and moderate and severe chronic shift work sleep disorder (Torrex Chiesi Polska Sp. z.o.o. 2008). Thus, excessive sleepiness associated with the listed chronic diseases was the only medical indication for prescribing the drug to the patient. The drug was not approved for enhancing cognitive powers in healthy individuals. Such an off-label use would be medically unjustified due to the lack of sufficient scientific evidence for favorable risk-benefit profile. Therefore, neither in the time when Vigil was on the Polish market, nor today, Jane's decision not to take modafinil could be judged as being contrary to the law governing her profession or the physician's duty of due care. On the contrary, a Polish physician or pharmacist who would prescribe or sell her the drug could be accused for acting illegally. The sole fact that in the Jane's hospital it was a common practice among surgeons to take smart drugs in order to stay on duty longer does not suffice to consider her decision reckless or negligent.

4.2. Is there an adequate causal link between Jane's decision and Richard's injuries?

As mentioned earlier, the Polish civil law adopts the principle of adequate causation which limits a tortfeasor's liability to normal consequences of her harmful conduct. In order to establish the scope of the tortfeasor's liability, the *conditio sine qua non* test and the assessment of the "normality" of the harmful effect (damage) are performed. In the case of Jane, the first test requires to determine whether Richard would have not suffered the injury if Jane had taken modafinil. The causal link between the injury and the Jane's decision is indirect – it is mediated by the erroneous conduct of the surgeon. Thus, the necessary causal links must be established:

(i) between Jane's decision to perform the surgery, when fatigued, without modafinil and the committed medical error, and (ii) between the error and the injury suffered by the patient. Unfortunately, the facts of the case as well as available scientific data on modafinil's efficacy do not allow for a definite determination of the necessary causations. Firstly, it is unknown whether indeed the injury occurred because Jane made a fatigue-related error. Although fatigue is one of the most common causes of medical errors (Bari et al. 2016), there are various other factors which lead to them, for example, incompetence, lack of proper knowledge or skills, inadequate experience, inadequate supervision, rush, lack of ordinary carefulness, etc. Secondly, even if it would be possible to establish that the patient's injury occurred in result of June's fatigue, scientific research show at best that modafinil has *some* beneficial effects on *selected* cognitive processes in *some* healthy but sleep-deprived individuals. However, these results do not support the conclusion that the drug eliminates all the effects of fatigue, and - what is the most important - that, if taken by Jane, it would have prevented the harmful fatigue-related error (Goold and Maslen 2014b). Thirdly, since the nature of Richard's injury and the nature of Jane's error are unknown, little can be said about causal relation between these two events. In summary, there is no ground for Richard to claim that if Jane had used modafinil, with the high degree of probability, she would not have committed the medical error and the injury would not have occurred. The necessary causal link between her omission, the error and the damage suffered by Richard cannot be definitely established.

Although the negative result of the *conditio sine qua non* test makes any further analysis of the causation void, for the sake of argument, we will proceed with the assessment of "normality" of the causal relations in question. Does Richard's injury fall within the range of "normal" consequence of Jane's decision to perform brain surgery without modafinil? Since the causal link between the damage and Jane's decision is indirect, the question needs to be divided in two:

- Does the probability of a fatigue-related medical error (similar to the one committed by Jane) significantly decrease each time a surgeon (with a specialization, qualifications, and experience similar to Jane's) takes modafinil?
- Does the probability of an injury (similar to the one experienced by Richard) significantly increase each time a surgeon makes a fatigue-related medical error (of a kind similar to the one committed by Jane)?

As argued above, the second question cannot be answered due to the lack of information on the nature of the Richard's injury as well as the nature of the medical error committed by Jane. An answer to the first questions depends on the scientific evidence, which is not conclusive. Firstly, although it is commonly believed that people in general and physicians in particular perform worse when they are sleep-deprived or fatigued, this conviction enjoys limited empirical support. Some studies have shown that sleepiness and fatigue affect cognitive and motor performance (Pilcher and Huffcutt 1996) and have negative impact on patient's safety (Baldwin and Daugherty 2004; West et al. 2009; Bari et al. 2016). But a systematic review of studies on the effects of fatigue on surgeons' performance and surgical outcomes – also quoted by Goold and Maslen (2014b, 435) – concludes that "the overall weight of (poor) evidence shows that clinical performance is not proven to be affected by sleep deprivation or fatigue and that psychomotor performance may or may not be" (Sturm et al. 2011, 508). Secondly, what has been already stressed, it is far from clear that pharmacological cognitive enhancers, such as modafinil, could indeed eliminate or correct cognitive impairments which are responsible for the alleged worse psychomotoric performance of fatigued individuals (Sugden at al. 2012). In sum, in the light of the current knowledge, it cannot be argued that the damage suffered by Richard in result of the error committed by Jane is a "normal" consequence of Jane's failure to take modafinil.

Conclusion

The case of Jane, an overworked and exhausted surgeon who has decided to complete her professional tasks without modafinil, provides a good example of new legal challenges that come with the development of cognitive enhancement technology. The authors of the scenario – Goold and Maslen – have analysed the case through the lens of a common law system – English tort law and case law (2014b). They have argued that in such cases, claims of negligence for a failure to enhance would be unlikely to succeed in English courts. We have come to a similar conclusion. Our analysis has shown that also in the Polish tort law claims in negligence against medical professionals for injuries, allegedly caused by a failure to use cognitive enhancers, are unlikely to succeed. Presently, there is no ground to claim that by refusing to take modafinil or other neuro-enhancing substance, a professional acts wrongfully (faulty) or in breach of her duty of due care.

Moreover, even if this could be established in the future, it would be very difficult to prove that there is an adequate causal link between the physician's failure to enhance and the patient's damage.

Acknowledgement

This analysis was funded by the Ministry of Science and Higher Education, Poland, Diamentowy Grant (Diamond Grant) No. DI2015006045.

Literature

Bączyk-Rozwadowska, K. (2011), Medical malpractice and compensation in Poland, *Chicago-Kent Law Review* 86, 1217–1261.

Bagińska, E. (2011) Medical liability in Poland, in Koch, B.A. (Ed) *Medical Liability in Europe. A Comparison of Selected Jurisdiction* (Tort and Insurance Law, vol. 29), Berlin-Boston: De Gruyter, 411–450.

Bagińska, E. (2013) Causal uncertainty and proportional liability in Poland, in Gilead, I, Green, M.D. and Koch, B.A. (Eds) *Proportional Liability: Analytical and Comparative Perspectives* (Tort and Insurance Law, vol. 33), Berlin-Boston: De Gruyter, 253–282.

Bagińska, E. and Tulibacka M. (2014) *Tort Law in Poland*, Wolters Kluwer Law & Business.

Baldwin Jr, D. C. and Daugherty, S. R. (2004) Sleep deprivation and fatigue in residency training: results of a national survey of first-and second-year residents, *Sleep* 27(2), 217–223.

Bari, A., Khan, R. A. and Rathore, A. W. (2016), Medical error: causes, consequences, emotional response and resulting behavioral change, *Pakistan Journal of Medical Sciences* 32(3), 523–528.

Bostrom, N. and Sandberg, A. (2009) Cognitive enhancement: methods, ethics, regulatory challenges, *Science and Engineering Ethics* 15(3), 311–341.

Bostrom, N. and Roache, R. (2011) Smart policy: cognitive enhancement in the public interest, in Savulescu, J., ter Meulen R. and Kahane, G. (Eds) *Enhancing Human Capacities*, Oxford: Wiley-Blackwell, 138–149.

Caldwell, J.A. (2005) Dextroamphetamine and modafinil are effective countermeasures for fatigue in the operational environment, in *Strategies to Maintain Combat Readiness During Extended Deployments – A Human Systems Approach*. Meeting Proceedings RTO-MP-HFM-124, Neuilly-sur-Seine, France: RTO, 31, 1–16, available online: http://www.rto.nato.int/abstracts.asp. (Access: 14.06.2017)

Caldwell, J. A., Caldwell, J. L., Smith, J. K. and Brown, D. L. (2004) Modafinil's effects on simulator performance and mood in pilots during 37 h without sleep, *Aviation, Space, and Environmental Medicine* 75(9), 777–784.

Chandler, J. A. (2013) Autonomy and the unintended legal consequences of emerging neurotherapies, *Neuroethics* 6(2), 249–263.

Coffman, B. A., Clark, V. P. and Parasuraman, R. (2014) Battery powered thought: enhancement of attention, learning, and memory in healthy adults using transcranial direct current stimulation, *Neuroimage* 85, 895–908.

de Sio, F. S., Faulmüller, N. and Vincent, N. A. (2014) How cognitive enhancement can change our duties, *Frontiers in Systems Neuroscience* 8, 131, available online: https://doi.org/10.3389/fnsys.2014.00131 (Access: 14.06.2017)

European Medicines Agency, EMA (2010), Modafinil, available online: http://www.ema.europa.eu/ema/index.jsp?curl=pages/medicines/human/referrals/Modafinil/human_referral_000236.jsp (Access: 14.06.2017)

Gill, M., Haerich, P., Westcott, K., Godenick, K. L. and Tucker, J. A. (2006) Cognitive performance following modafinil versus placebo in sleep-deprived emergency physicians: a double blind randomized crossover study, *Academic Emergency Medicine* 13(2), 158–165.

Goold, I. and Maslen, H. (2014a) Must the surgeon take the pill? Negligence duty in the context of cognitive enhancement, *The Modern Law Review* 77(1), 60–86.

Goold, I. and Maslen, H. (2014b) Obliging surgeons to enhance: negligence liability for uncorrected fatigue and problems with proving causation, *Medical Law Review* 23(3), 427–454.

Goold, I., and Maslen, H. (2015) Responsibility enhancement and the law of negligence, in Clausen, J., and Levy, N. (Eds) *Handbook of Neuroethics*, Dordrecht:Springer Netherlands, 1363–1380.

Grady, S., Aeschbach, D., Wright, K. P. and Czeisler, C. A. (2010) Effect of modafinil on impairments in neurobehavioral performance and learning associated with extended wakefulness and circadian misalignment, *Neuropsychopharmacology* 35(9), 1910–1920.

Hart, C. L., Haney, M., Vosburg, S. K., Comer, S. D., Gunderson, E. and Foltin, R. W. (2006) Modafinil attenuates disruptions in cognitive performance during simulated night-shift work, *Neuropsychopharmacology* 31(7), 1526–1536.

Hildt, E. and Franke, A.G. (2013) *Cognitive Enhancement. An Interdisciplinary Perspective*, Dordrecht: Springer.

Housden, C.R., Morein-Zamir, S. and Sahakian, B.J. (2011) Cognitive enhancing drugs: neuroscience and society, in Savulescu, J., ter Meulen R. and Kahane, G. (Eds) *Enhancing Human Capacities*, Oxford: Wiley-Blackwell, 113–126.

Jotterand, F. and Dubljevic, V. (2016) *Cognitive Enhancement: Ethical and Policy Implications in International Perspective*, London: Oxford University Press.

Kalus, S. (2009) Liability for medical damages in Polish law, in Heiderhoff, B. and Żmij, G. (Eds) *Tort Law in Poland, Germany and Europe*, Munich: Sellier European Law Publishers, 48–74.

Klimesch, W., Sauseng, P. and Gerloff, C. (2003) Enhancing cognitive performance with repetitive transcranial magnetic stimulation at human individual alpha frequency, *European Journal of Neuroscience* 17(5), 1129–1133.

Koch, A. (1975) *Związek przyczynowy jako podstawa odpowiedzialności odszkodowawczej w prawie cywilnym* [Causal Link as a Basic Condition for Compensatory Liability in the Civil Law], Warsaw: Państwowe Wydawnictwo Naukowe.

Müller, U., Rowe, J. B., Rittman, T., Lewis, C., Robbins, T. W. and Sahakian, B. J. (2013) Effects of modafinil on non-verbal cognition, task enjoyment and creative thinking in healthy volunteers, *Neuropharmacology* 64, 490–495.

Nesterowicz, M. (2013) *Prawo medyczne* [Medical Law] 10th Ed., Toruń: Dom Organizatora TNOiK.

Pilcher, J. J and Huffcutt, A. I. (1996) Effects of sleep deprivation on performance: a meta-analysis, *Sleep* 19(4), 318–326.

Randall, D. C., Shneerson, J. M. and File, S. E. (2005), Cognitive effects of modafinil in student volunteers may depend on IQ, *Pharmacology Biochemistry and Behavior* 82(1), 133–139.

Randall, D. C., Shneerson, J. M., Plaha, K. K. and File, S. E. (2003), Modafinil affects mood, but not cognitive function, in healthy young volunteers, *Human Psychopharmacology: Clinical and Experimental* 18(3), 163–173.

Republic of Poland, Act of 23rd April 1964 – Civil Code [Kodeks Cywilny], *Journal of Laws [Dziennik Ustaw]* Dz.U. 2018, pos. 1025 with further amendments (consolidated text).

Republic of Poland, Act of 5th December 1996 on the Professions of Physician and Dentist [*ustawa o zawodach lekarza i lekarza dentysty*], *Journal of Laws [Dziennik Ustaw]* Dz.U. 2018, pos. 617 with further amendments (consolidated text).

Richmond, L. L., Wolk, D., Chein, J. and Olson, I. R. (2014) Transcranial direct current stimulation enhances verbal working memory training performance over time and near transfer outcomes, *Journal of Cognitive Neuroscience* 26(11), 2443–2454.

Sandberg, A. (2011) Cognition enhancement: upgrading the brain, in Savulescu, J., ter Meulen R. and Kahane, G. (Eds) *Enhancing Human Capacities*, Oxford: Wiley-Blackwell, 71–91.

Sandberg, A. and Savulescu J., (2011) The social and economic impacts of cognitive enhancement, in Savulescu, J., ter Meulen R. and Kahane, G. (Eds) *Enhancing Human Capacities*, Oxford: Wiley-Blackwell, 92–112.

Sturm, L., Dawson, D., Vaughan, R., Hewett, P., Hill, A. G., Graham, J. C. and Maddern, G. J. (2011), Effects of fatigue on surgeon performance and surgical outcomes: a systematic review, *ANZ Journal of Surgery* 81(7–8), 502–509.

Sugden, C., Housden, C. R., Aggarwal, R., Sahakian, B. J. and Darzi, A. (2012) Effect of pharmacological enhancement on the cognitive and clinical psychomotor performance of sleep-deprived doctors: a randomized controlled trial, *Annals of Surgery* 255(2), 222–227.

Torrex Chiesi Polska Sp.z.o.o (2008) *Komunikat dla osób wykonujących zawód medyczny dotyczący związku między preparatem Vigil (Modafinilum) a ciężką wysypką i zaburzeniami psychicznymi [Information for Medical Professionals on the Relationship between Vigil and Severe Rush and Psychiatric Disorders*], available online: http://www.leki-informacje.pl/sites/default/files/bezpieczenstwo/vigil.pdf. (Access: 14.06.2017)

Torrex Chiesi Polska Sp.z.o.o (2011) *Powiadomienie o stałym wstrzymaniu obrotu produktem leczniczym* [*Notification on the Permanent Marketing Suspension of a Medicinal Product*], available online: http://www.dia.com.pl/download/3667/ (Access: 14.06.2017)

Turner, D. C., Robbins, T. W., Clark, L., Aron, A. R., Dowson, J. and Sahakian, B. J. (2003) Cognitive enhancing effects of modafinil in healthy volunteers, *Psychopharmacology* 165(3), 260–269.

U.S. Food and Drug Administration, FDA (1998), *Drug Approval Package: Provigil (Modafinil) Tablets*, avaliable online: https://www.accessdata.fda.gov/drugsatfda_docs/nda/98/020717A_Provigil.cfm. (Access: 14.06.2017)

Vincent, N. (2011) The challenges posed to private law by emerging cognitive enhancement technologies, in Muller S., Zouridis S., Frishman M. and Kistemaker L. (Eds) *The Law of the Future and The Future of Law*, Oslo: Torkel Opsahl Academic EPublisher, 511–521, available online: http://www.fichl.org/fileadmin/fichl/documents/FICHL_11_Web.pdf. (Access: 14.06.2017)

Vincent, N. (2013) Enhancing responsibility, in Vincent, N. (Ed) *Neuroscience and Legal Responsibility*, New York, NY: Oxford University Press: 305–333.

Vlek, R. J., Steines, D., Szibbo, D., Kübler, A., Schneider, M. J., Haselager, P. and Nijboer, F. (2012) Ethical issues in brain-computer interface research, development, and dissemination, *Journal of Neurologic Physical Therapy* 36(2), 94–99.

West, C.P., Tan, A.D., Habermann, T.M., Sloan, J.A. and Shanafelt, T.D. (2009) Association of resident fatigue and distress with perceived medical errors, *JAMA* 302(12), 1294–1300.

Zimerman, M. and Hummel, F. C. (2010) Non-invasive brain stimulation: enhancing motor and cognitive functions in healthy old subjects, *Frontiers in Aging Neuroscience* 2, 149, available online: http://journal.frontiersin.org/article/10.3389/fnagi.2010.00149/full. (Access: 14.06.2017)

Żmij, G. (2009) Wrongfulness as a liability's prerequisite in art 415 Polish Civil Code, in Heiderhoff, B. and Żmij, G. (Eds) *Tort Law in Poland, Germany and Europe*, Munich : Sellier European Law Publishers, 13–22.

List of Contributors

Gabriel Bianchi, Associate Professor, Institute for Research in Social Communication, Slovak Academy of Sciences, Bratislava, Slovakia

Andrzej Girdwoyń, MJur, Center for Bioethics and Biolaw, University of Warsaw, Warsaw, Poland

Josef Kuře, Associate Professor, Department of Medical Ethics, Faculty of Medicine, Masaryk University, Brno, Czech Republic

Juraj Odorčák, Juraj Odorčák, PhD, Department of Philosophy and Applied Philosophy, Faculty of Arts, University of Sts. Cyril and Methodius, Trnava, Slovakia

Ivars Neiders, Associate Professor, Department of Humanities, Rīga, Stradiņš University, Riga, Latvia

Miroslav Popper, Associate Professor, Institute for Research in Social Communication, Slovak Academy of Sciences, Bratislava, Slovakia

Emil Višňovský, Professor, Institute for Research in Social Communication, Slovak Academy of Sciences, Bratislava, Slovakia

Joanna Różyńska, PhD, Center for Bioethics and Biolaw, University of Warsaw, Warsaw, Poland

Peter Sýkora, Professor, Centre for Bioethics, Department of Philosophy and Applied Philosophy, Faculty of Arts, University of Sts. Cyril and Methodius, Trnava, Slovakia

Jana Tomašovičová, PhD, Department of Philosophy and Applied Philosophy, Faculty of Arts, University of Sts. Cyril and Methodius, Trnava, Slovakia

Index

FSC
www.fsc.org
MIX
Papier | Fördert
gute Waldnutzung
FSC® C083411

Kolibri 360 GmbH
Ferdinand-Jühlke-Straße 7
99095 Erfurt, Deutschland
produktsicherheit@kolibri360.de